Lessons from Joan

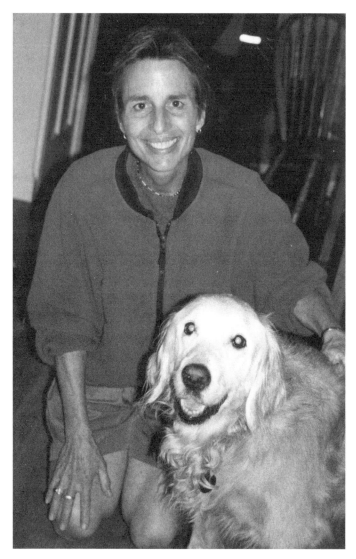

Joan and Baltimore, 2000.

Lessons from Joan

Living and Loving with Cancer, A Husband's Story

Eric R. Kingson

With a Foreword by Karen Davis

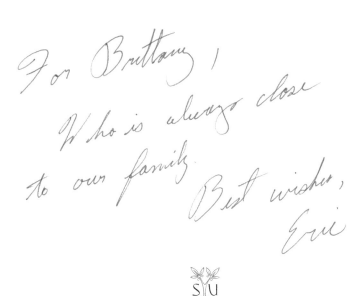

For Brittany,
Who is always close
to our family. Best wishes,
Eric

SYRACUSE UNIVERSITY PRESS

First Edition 2005
06 07 08 09 00   6 5 4 3 2

All photographs courtesy of the author except where indicated.
The author gratefully acknowledges the permission to reprint excerpts from the following texts:

in chapter 6: "Autumn Rose Elegy," from *The Glance: Rumi's Songs of Soul-Meeting* by Rumi, translated by Coleman Barks, copyright © 1999 by Coleman Barks. Used by permission of Viking Penguin, a division of Penguin Group (USA) Inc.

in chapter 7: Excerpt of "In Blackwater Woods," from *American Primitive* by Mary Oliver. Copyright © 1978, 1979, 1980, 1981, 1982, 1983 by Mary Oliver. By permission of Little, Brown and Co., Inc.

in appendix B: Y. Fong, L. H. Blumgart, and A. M. Cohen, "Surgical Treatment of Colorectal Metastases to the Liver, "*CA: Cancer Journal for Clinicians* 45, no. 1 (Jan.–Feb. 1995): 50–62. Reprinted with permission of Lippincott Williams & Wilkins.

Y. Fong, N. Kemeny, P. Paty, L. H. Blumgart, and A. M. Cohen, "Treatment of Colorectal Cancer: Hepatic Metastasis," *Seminars in Surgical Oncology* 12, no. 4 (July–Aug. 1996): 219–52. Copyright © 1996. Reprinted with permission of Wiley-Liss, Inc., a subsidiary of John Wiley & Sons, Inc.

Nancy Kemeny, Ying Huang, Alfred M. Cohen, Weiji Shi, John A. Conti, Murray F. Brennan, Joseph R. Bertino, Alan D. M. Turnbull, Deirdre Sullivan, Jennifer Stockman, Leslie H. Blumgart, and Yuman Fong, "Hepatic Arterial Infusion of Chemotherapy after Resection of Hepatic Metastases from Colorectal Cancer," *New England Journal of Medicine* 341 (1999): 2039–48. Copyright © 1999 Massachusetts Medical Society. All rights reserved.

The paper used in this publication meets the minimum requirements of American National Standard for Information Sciences—Permanence of Paper for Printed Library Materials, ANSI Z39.48–1984.∞™

Library of Congress Cataloging-in-Publication Data
Kingson, Eric R.
Lessons from Joan : living and loving with cancer, a husband's story / Eric R. Kingson, with a foreword by Karen Davis.— 1st ed.
p. cm.
ISBN 0–8156–0838–1 (alk. paper)
1. Kingson, Joan, 1951– Health. 2. Cancer—Patients—Biography. 3. Cancer—Patients—Family relationships. I. Title.
RC265.6.K56K56 2005
362.196'994'0092—dc22   2005022072

To Joan, with love

To Aaron and Johanna, with love

To Cathy and George, with love

To Susan and Scott Plumb,
who walked a similar path with grace

To Dr. Nancy Kemeny, Dr. Tony Scalzo,
and those who cared for Joan,
with appreciation

And for all who give of themselves
in care for others

The author's proceeds from the sale of this book will be used to support efforts that give expression to the values of care to which Joan was committed in her work with children and families. An annual award has been established to recognize a Crouse Hospital service or technical worker whose special interactions with patients and families vividly reflect these values:

Treating each patient as an individual

Respecting patients' social, emotional, intellectual, spiritual, and physical needs

Welcoming families, especially the young, into the caring process

Enhancing patient understanding of procedures and choices

Listening

Contents

Illustrations

Foreword

KAREN DAVIS

ᒫ Joan's experience with the health care system has lessons for all of us. Most importantly, it illustrates the importance of "the heart" in our health care system—for our patients, family members, health care providers, and our culture. Care is more than accessing the best technology and physicians, though obviously good technical medicine is very important. When health care is tilted too much toward efficiency and delivering care in measured units, everyone is diminished.

Conversely, care that incorporates and engages the hearts of patients, families, and people who provide care can be—regardless of outcomes—strengthening of everyone involved and reinforcing of important societal values including the promotion of dignity and respect for our common humanity.

Joan was fortunate to have a loving and tireless advocate for her

Karen Davis is president of the Commonwealth Fund, a national philanthropy engaged in independent research on health and social policy issues. A nationally recognized economist, she served as deputy assistant secretary for health policy in the Department of Health and Human Services from 1977–1980, making her the first woman to head a U.S. public health service agency. Ms. Davis is author of several landmark books on health policy including *Health Care Cost Containment; Medicare Policy; National Health Insurance: Benefits, Costs, and Consequences;* and *Health and the War on Poverty.* She was selected to the Institute of Medicine in 1975 and has served two terms on its governing council (1986–1990 and 1997–2000).

care. Eric not only provided essential emotional support but helped her research care options and, when necessary, was willing to go to bat to clear the obstacles to getting the care that improved her quality of life and gave her extra time with her family and friends. However, at a time when their full focus should have been on Joan's health and their family, it is unfortunate that dealing with billing and coverage concerns about insurance were excessively time consuming and often draining.

Joan brought out the best in those around her, and this undoubtedly contributed to the quality of her care. She was an exceptionally decent and engaging person. It was clear to providers that she was doing everything she could to live as long as possible and that, in spite of everything, she was appreciative of the extra life she was getting. And she was genuinely appreciative of the care she received—whether by physicians, nurses, aides, or other personnel.

But she also had many strengths that aren't available to all families. She had excellent health care coverage, and, in spite of hassles with insurance providers and medical billing offices, for the most part she was able to get what she needed and was treated with courtesy. And, while it might have been a strain, she and Eric could afford to cover what wasn't paid for. She knew how to marshal information, engage others, and advocate for the type of care she needed. Many health professionals could identify with her as a middle-class mother, professional educator, and nurse. She gravitated toward health care professionals who listened to and respected their patients. Eric had flexibility in his job and good colleagues willing to help with his load. Finally, and very importantly, Joan's children, sisters, brother, and other family members and friends were very present and supportive throughout her illness. Joan had much guidance from friends with professional knowledge of the health care system who helped her navigate a complex and often confusing system.

Some lessons to be drawn from Joan's experience are that:

People should not have to be "consumer-savvy," upper-middle-class professionals to get the services they need. Joan was acutely aware of huge inequities in our society and our health care system. Her experience was clearly different from that of many others who also face extremely difficult diagnoses. That contrast—between what she received versus what, for example, an isolated older person or someone without health insurance or her education is likely to receive—should not be accepted as "just the way it is."

Patient/family-centered care is important. Medical, nursing, and other health care professionals' training should emphasize the significance of listening to and of engaging the family in care. There is a related need for health care professionals to receive education on the importance of working with family members/advocates in the treatment process and in providing patient-centered care. This is especially essential in the face of financial pressures on health care institutions and the pressure to extract "inefficiencies" out of the health care system.

Health care systems need to provide and/or encourage patients to bring an "advocate." Patients with a life-threatening illness and their families are often scared and overwhelmed. More should be done to assist patients in dealing with the health care system when faced with a frightening diagnosis. Patient navigators are being tried in some hospitals to good effect. This model should spread more widely, and reimbursement for patient navigator services would propel this movement. Patients also need tools like decision-making videos to help them think through choices.

We need to encourage and reward health care providers for taking the time to engage the humanity of their patients and their families. Many do take that time, of course, but our health care system often makes doing so difficult. Besides excellent medicine and nursing care, what is most important to patients and their families are many small acts of kindness. Feedback from patients, through patient-centered care surveys or other means, is an important step in improving care that is responsive to patient and family needs. Any system of "pay for performance" rewards should also incorporate patients' reports on care experiences.

Patients should have quick access to test results. Long waits for test results are a source of great anxiety for many people undergoing treatment. In an information-driven society, it should be possible to provide quick access to such information.

Oncologists and other treating professionals should be trained about the importance of maintaining contact with patients and families during the dying process. Joan was fortunate to have caring and professional end-of-life care. But patients often report feeling abandoned by their oncologists when it becomes clear that their condition is no longer treatable.

Good health care requires engaging the humanity of patients, families, and providers. Health care is not just about the physical. It should also be concerned with the emotional and spiritual well-being of patients, their families, and even of people giving the care.

None of us knows when serious illness will strike our families. Learning from the experiences of others can be invaluable in shaping public policy and health care practice. By learning from stories such as Joan's, we can help make certain that the kind of care we need and want will be there for us. Most importantly, it will help us have a health care system that truly is a leader in ensuring patient-centered care not just for those who can work the system but for those who are most vulnerable in the face of serious illness.

Lessons from Joan

1

Endings and the Start of the Story

May 13, 2001

Dear Friends,

Joan found a peaceful death early yesterday morning—forty-three years, to the day, after her mother died. In the past few days, she expressed a couple of times that she was feeling the presence of her mother. After caring for others so well, we hope she is in her mother's arms.

She truly was not afraid of dying. She expressed many times that given the progression of the cancer, she saw death as a release from, as she put it, "this bag of bones" and as a welcomed transition to a different place. She and I were asleep in the hospital room when she died. My hands were resting on her chest and head.

A few days ago, Joan asked that all treatment, including hydration and nutrition, be stopped and that things only be done to keep her pain free and comfortable.

She and I and our family are very grateful for the exceptionally kind and competent nursing and medical care she received for thirty-one days on the fourth floor of Syracuse's Crouse Hospital.

Aaron, Johanna, and I and the rest of the family are as okay as we can be after this kind of loss. I am deeply sad but could not have asked for a better life with her, only much longer.

Words from one of the closing songs from *Les Misérables* keep coming to mind:

> Take my hand and lead me to salvation
> Take my love, for love is everlasting
> And remember the truth that once was spoken
> To love another person is to see the face of God

On a more practical side, for those who are able to come I am including information about the funeral arrangements and directions to our home. We will hold the funeral service at 1:00 P.M. on Wednesday, May 16 in the backyard of our home at 8278 Glen Eagle Drive, Manlius, New York, followed by her burial at Oakwood Cemetery in Syracuse. We are inviting anyone who wishes to join us back at our home for an informal dinner and time to enjoy each other and the memory of Joan.

Joan, as you know, was a pretty informal person. In keeping with the way we think she would want things done, we want to encourage you to dress comfortably. No need for ties or dark clothes, etc., but of course you are welcome to wear whatever feels right to you.

For those who may wish to come but are unable to do so, please know that we consider the kindnesses and feelings between you and Joan and our family in life to be what is most important, not whether you're able to attend the funeral. So, our friends, you are very welcome, but do not feel you need to turn yourself into a pretzel to be here for this one moment. It is the other moments that are most important.

Warmly and with appreciation,
Eric

I take great pride in the memory of our love and in the way Joan, I, and our children, Aaron and Johanna, handled the thirty-two months that followed Joan's cancer diagnosis.

In many ways, we did everything right. Joan faced the disease with courage, driven in part by her determination to maintain our home in the face of a devastating illness. Our children adjusted to and thrived in a new school and community. I settled into a new job. Our love grew stronger. Our families and friends were wonderful. Joan's older sister, Catherine Fernbach, traveled from Boston to our home outside Syracuse every two to three weeks. George Igel, a lifelong friend and psychiatrist, guided us through many health decisions. Time took on special meaning. We enjoyed our lives together.

We sought and received exceptional health care, developing trusting and warm relationships with the doctors, nurses, social workers, aides, secretaries, and many others involved in Joan's care. We were well informed. We gained access to state-of-the-art treatments for metastatic colon cancer. Our health insurance paid the bills. We didn't go broke.

Many people benefited from our experience. With rare exception, Joan did not retreat into herself, angry and depressed. She maintained genuine interest in family, friends, and new acquaintances. In her final weeks in the hospital, she spoke with the nurses and aides about their own children and educational experiences. With impish humor, she told my boss that she would not be able to "die in peace" unless he hired a professional friend she greatly respected. She videotaped messages for our children, her sister Catherine, and me. She did not wish to die, but she did not see death as an awful event, to be avoided at all costs (as if any of us can). I learned from Joan, along with many others, that death does not require terror, not even fear, and that it can be a release, though I would be hard pressed to call it a "friend" from the vantage point of someone who survived the loss of a beloved spouse.

The little child part of me asks, why, given that we did virtually everything right, did it turn out this way? What went wrong? Why did Joan have to die, twenty-two years into our marriage, leaving our sixteen-year-old daughter, Johanna, and nineteen-year-old son, Aaron? Why did she leave me? Why didn't God intervene?

So far, I have had only one satisfying—admittedly only partially satisfying—answer to my queries. Perhaps everything happened the way it did *because* we did everything right. Perhaps Joan died peacefully in my arms because we did everything right. Perhaps she lived two years more than she should have because . . . Perhaps my and our children's grief is so intense because . . .

A corollary of this may be, imagine just how bad things would have been if we hadn't done everything right!

I do not know the answer to the "why" questions. I do not know why this disease found Joan; why she is not here; why I and my children are deprived of her physical presence.

But I am certain that Joan's capacity to grow and to maintain dignity, wisdom, and humor carry meaning. And I hope to convey this meaning to those dealing with similarly life-threatening illnesses—either as patients, family members, friends, or health care providers.

This book is about how we dealt with Joan's illness, and the fear, hope, and intensity of our lives during the thirty-two months that followed her diagnosis. It's about how Joan and I and our children maintained a good family life during this time and the importance of love shown by family and friends. It's about some of the funny things that happened along the way. It's about lessons learned from other patients and the value of everyday kindnesses of secretaries, health care providers, parking lot attendants, fellow patients, and others.

This book is also about what we did to access compassionate, state-of-the-art care. It's about aggressive interventions that provided hope and improved the quality of Joan's life. It's about how we researched options, and how we worked with health care providers in making difficult choices. It's about how we presented our questions on one page in advance of meetings with doctors, how we crafted letters to gain approval from our insurance company for participation in clinical trials.

While mindful that access to quality care for all remains a shamefully distant dream in our nation, this book is about how the health care system worked on our behalf. It's about hospitals that provided good care; about oncologists, surgeons, nurses, and highly specialized researchers who gave of themselves to Joan and others; about the extraordinary demands on and care provided by the great majority of the floor nurses, doctors, nurses aides, and social workers with whom we had contact (and about how we avoided some of the others).

Most centrally, this book is about living and dying with dignity, hope, and humor. And how doing so enriches many lives and helps with the healing of those left behind.

This is not the book I hoped to write. In fact, I didn't plan on writing one at all. If I had, I would have wanted to write about how Joan's healthy spirit and strong will to live and our careful research and selection of physicians and interventions resulted in remission and cure.

And when Joan was diagnosed, this is not the type of book we turned to first. We would have been interested in some of the practical advice you'll find in this book, especially in appendix A, which summarizes the lessons gleaned from our experience. We would have been interested in the examples presented in the appendices of the letters and memos we used to communicate with physicians and insurers and to seek information about state-of-the-art care. But mostly we wanted to read about how people "beat cancer," about cures against great odds or about how cancer could become a chronic illness. Only later in our journey might we have been interested in learning about how people lived with cancer and the approach of death.

Besides sorting through the pain and deep loss we experienced, I hope to provide a road map for those that follow. I believe there are lessons for everyday life—mine and yours—and for families and friends facing similar illnesses.

Many who read this book will be in the midst of their own struggles with cancer or other life-threatening illnesses. I wish each of you many years of good health and happiness. May you find some of what you need—including a laugh or two—to continue to grow and thrive with strength and love of life on your own journey, wherever it leads.

Other readers will be the close family and friends of people experiencing illnesses such as Joan's. I hope the pages that follow provide further support, recognition, and reason for satisfaction in the care you are giving to those you love.

Still others will be students and providers of professional care. I hope this book provides you with useful insight into the experiences of your patients and their families. As you read through its pages, I hope you will find satisfaction in the gratitude that patients and family feel for competently and kindly given care that respects and gives expression to the dignity of each patient and to their connections to life, no matter how ill.

Notwithstanding the death of the protagonist of this story, I believe you will find that this is a fundamentally optimistic story, including the epilogue, which talks about life after cancer.

I begin with our lives before.

2

Beginnings

Joan and I "had" (I still feel "have") a very good marriage.

We had our differences.

I am sloppy. She is neat. I organize myself horizontally with piles of papers and things left everywhere. Joan organized herself (and sometimes me) vertically, papers carefully placed in files. A sometimes not insignificant source of marital tension, Joan often insisted on putting my papers—sometimes strewn all over the dining room table or anywhere else I might be working—into tidy piles.

For a while, I thought that one of the "worse" things about her death was that I no longer had someone to blame when my books, lecture notes, electronic organizer, or shoes wandered from where I had left them.

Joan's neatness was very much a part of her—enough so that our close friends sometimes joked about it. An example: as Joan approached death, we discussed places for burial, narrowing the choice down to a well-manicured versus a "well-charactered" cemetery in close proximity to my work. In discussing my preference for the latter with Joan's close friend Michele Melville, I said that it was "very nice, a bit funky and not 100 percent neat." Michele commented, "Sounds perfect; it will give Joan something to clean up at night." In reflecting on Michele's comment, I now realize that Joan's penchant for an orderly home is not confined by death. Indeed, not only is she straightening up Oakwood

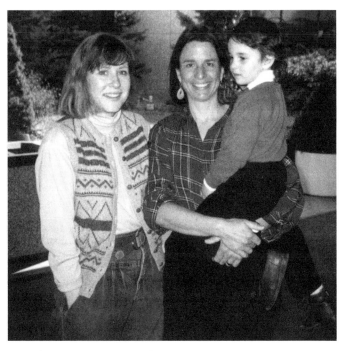

Good friends: Michele Melville, Joan, and Johanna, 1986.

Cemetery, but, to my dismay, she continues to organize my life and papers. How else could I explain so many mysterious disappearances?

I am a sprinter; Joan a steady long-distance runner. I procrastinate, but once I get started (which isn't as much as I would like), I often do not stop. I've written through many dinners and, when younger, often through the night, only stopping when I felt my work complete. I wasn't much around the house, but every once in a while I would work non-stop painting a porch, sanding the floors in our vacation home, installing a Rube Goldberg sump pump in the basement, putting a family celebration together. Joan, on the other hand, did a little (really, if the truth be told, a lot) every day—the laundry, the meals, household records, the photo albums, reviewing the kids' homework, the garden—all the things that made our day-to-day life wonderful. As Joan put it, she preferred to "chunk away at things."

I read about social policy; Joan reads novels.

I am Jewish; Joan was born Catholic.

I find motion, activity, and being around a lot of people a relaxing way to spend a vacation; Joan had greater tolerance for solitude.

I like to squeeze every second out of vacations; Joan liked to be home a day or two early to get the kids ready for school.

Normal Mars/Venus issues aside, we had a good and enjoyable love life.

Over time, we did a pretty good job of negotiating our differences. We shared much: commitment to our marriage and to building a family, respect and appreciation for each other, love and pride in our children, enjoyment of friends and family, attachment to our various pets—Francis, Solo, Leda, Stitches, Baltimore, and Billie. We loved summer time spent together in our Adirondack home—long walks (being something of a slug, I sometimes called them "death marches"), swimming holes, cookouts at Cascade Lake, auctions, fixing up our summer home, and, most centrally, the warmth and laughter that came from being together with our children, family, and friends. We enjoyed neighborhood and community life. We were involved in Aaron's and Johanna's schools. We coached soccer, and we found friendships in our neighborhoods. We chose not to affiliate in a traditional sense with a synagogue or church, but felt the presence of a spirit in our lives and home. Our children had beautiful bar and bat mitzvahs in our backyard. We found room in our home and hearts for Christmas and Hanukkah, Easter and Passover. And we loved to laugh.

Our commitment to marriage and children was intensified by losses sustained as children—she, her mother at age six and I, my father at age thirteen. She had to deal with her father's, and I with my mother's, emotional problems.

We saw work—my teaching, research, and social policy involvements and her teaching and direct service with children—as a vehicle for giving expression to our concern for others and our beliefs in the importance of access for all to excellent schools, health care, employment, and a decent place to live.

And we shared our love of just being together.

LIVES BEFORE EACH OTHER

Nothing in our early histories suggests that a good marriage and family were foreordained.

Joan's parents—Paul Fernbach and Eleanor Mudge—met and married in Brisbane, Australia, during the Second World War. Her father was stationed as a surgeon and her mother as a nurse. Paul had been raised by aunts and uncles in Buffalo and had very little contact with his parents. Eleanor's parents, from a "well-established" Protestant family in Baltimore, were not pleased with her marriage to a Catholic.

At war's end, the Fernbachs set up their home and Paul's vascular surgery practice in Buffalo, New York. Children followed quickly— Dennis, born in 1947, Catherine in 1949, Joan in 1951, and Mary Jo in 1954. Normalcy had returned to the country and so, it seemed, to the Fernbachs.

Unfortunately, harsher realities prevailed. Joan's father struggled with a drinking problem and what I suspect today would be recognized as depression. A very bright man and a good provider, he was considered an excellent and, I recall Joan telling me, compassionate doctor. His drinking, often out of control, created much uncertainty and embarrassment in his children's lives. But there were also good times with her father and Joan spoke with fondness about their walks.

Eleanor contracted polio in 1953. She struggled with paralysis and other effects of the disease for five years. A mother of three at the time of diagnosis, her fourth was born in an iron lung! Often, she was totally unable to care for herself.

Years later, as Joan dealt with her own illness, she would wonder how desperately hard it must have been for her mother with four children to care for, a failing body, and an emotionally dysfunctional husband. Joan was only six when her mother died. As an adult, she did not have many recollections of her mother, a source of sadness more than resentment. She did, however, have a tremendous drive to give her children what she had lacked—warm and consistent mothering—no matter what.

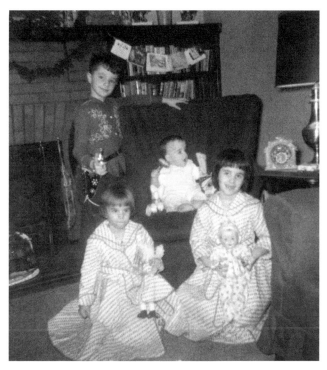

Dennis, Joan, Mary Jo, and Cathy: "the Fernbach kids," 1954.

Joan's father remarried. His new wife, Betty Buffum, the owner of a rat extermination business, lost both of her husbands to suicide—her first in 1964 and Paul in 1972. Losing their mother to polio was horrible for Joan and her siblings. But having Betty in their lives seems to have been still worse.

Consistent with her profession, her relationship with her stepchildren was poisonous. She thrived on laying emotional "traps" for her stepchildren, on berating each in turn. Family dinners became opportunities to expose and embarrass for the most minor of "infractions"—taking an extra cookie, using too much toilet paper. Outwardly a strong supporter of the ASPCA, Betty chose to put the family dog to death after Joan's father died, rather than allowing Cathy to take it to her Cambridge, Massachusetts, apartment. Cambridge was no place for a dog to

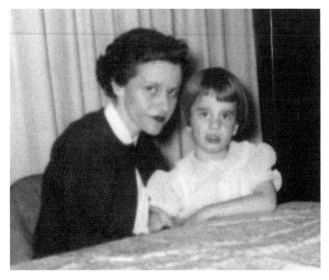

Joan and her mother, Eleanor Fernbach, 1956.

live! On hearing of Betty's death in 1975, Joan and Cathy—both very compassionate human beings—spontaneously broke out in song: "ding-dong, the witch is dead."

Betty's legacy is really quite remarkable. Whenever any of the Fernbachs get together, the discussion inevitably turns to how sadistic and undermining she was. In seeking to understand her cancer, Joan sometimes conceptualized it as "Betty," a malignancy best excised by surgery.

Joan's brother and sisters found strength and friendship, and normal rivalries, among themselves. Summer camp, beginning at very young ages, with Linda Butler (now Linda Butler Masters), their childhood friend and "fifth sibling" who lived across from them on Dorchester Road in Buffalo, was stabilizing and kindled Joan's love of the outdoors. Joan's aunt, Beth Fernbach, describes Joan as energetic, perhaps the hellion of the family, but also full of life, humor, and fun. She went to Catholic schools. A good student, she graduated as class president from the Nottingham School. The nuns at Nottingham—involved in the activist movements of the 1960s—made a lasting positive impression. And there were always good friends. Joan emerged from a painful childhood as a compassionate, caring, and competent young adult.

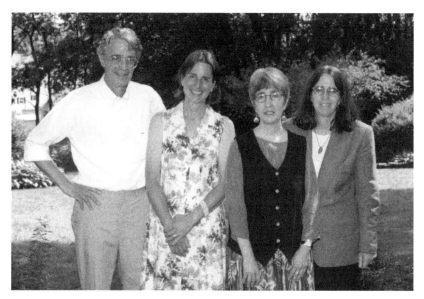

*Dennis, Joan, Cathy, and Mary Jo: "the Fernbach kids," 1998. Courtesy of
Judy Salsich.*

I don't really know much about Joan's college years at St. Lawrence
University, except that there were some periods of deep unhappiness.
After college, she held a couple of teaching positions in New Hamp-
shire, and she moved in 1973 to the Boston area, where she worked with
chronically ill children and later received a master's degree in special
education from Lesley College. There were some boyfriends, but none
that I know (or truthfully want to know) much about. And none as wonderful as me!

Born in 1946, I grew up in Manhattan, attending private schools, and
like many people from "The City," could not imagine wanting to live
anywhere else. My father, Milton Kingson, was the successful president
of Millburn Mills, a small textile firm. He liked to be in charge. As with
many men of his generation, his primary understanding of his role as a
family person was as a provider. And he was a good one. He was sixteen
years older than my mother, Ethel Schachtel, a beautiful woman. He
treated her more like an object than a partner, showering her with cloth-
ing and jewelry—not my approach to marriage, but one that was consis-

tent with the ethic of a "successful" male of his day. Friends and family remember his quickness of wit and temper. "He could be overbearing and patronizing, but it is also clear from stories and letters of condolence," as my mother wrote years later to Steve and me, "that he was loving, compassionate, and generous" and extremely active in several charities and his temple. "Mickey," she said, "loved me, his sons, his business, his golf and cards—in that order." I never had as much of him as I wanted, even when he was well, but I did feel cared for by him. He was diagnosed with colon cancer in 1954.

My mother, a kind woman, was crippled by depression, which I was told began when I was critically ill in 1948. My brother Steve, three years older than me, and I have too many memories of the months—sometimes as many as three in a row—she spent in bed deeply depressed. And of times defined as "feeling better" when she might be dusting in the middle of the night or be physically exhausted from excessive activity. As a child, teen, and even sometimes as an adult, I was embarrassed by what I viewed as her incompetence in negotiating the world, saddened by her suffering and angered by her needs.

My mother considered herself very fortunate to have two "dear, loving, caring parents" and a happy childhood. She wrote that her mother "was the Matriarch, the guiding force" and role model in her childhood family. Her father, a baker, "worked seven days a week for sixty years before he retired" and made what Albert Einstein—and many others who regularly purchased his ryes, challahs, and salt sticks—referred to as the best Jewish breads in America. "Growing up in a family of six children there was much teasing, lots of good cooking, good times and fun."

In hindsight and, in part, as a result of caring for Joan, I have a much better understanding of my mother's life accomplishments. For someone who suffered so much, it is remarkable that she never attempted suicide. She never gave up and always hoped to "lick this thing."

My mother was a deeply caring person. My childhood friends and others still comment about how nice she was. Her nephews and nieces remember her as always having time for them and never forgetting a

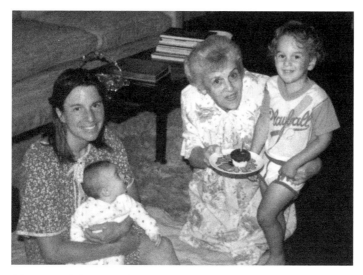

Johanna and Aaron, with Joan and their grandmother, Ethel Kingson, 1986.

birthday. Shortly before she died, she wrote, "One life is not enough for all the lessons there are to learn. Thank God for children and grandchildren! The love we receive we give away. I hope I may leave my sons and their children the legacy of my love. That is what really counts!" Indeed, she succeeded.

And, when my father was diagnosed with colon cancer in 1954, she used all her energy and love to continue their lives and care for him. Her way did not become the approach that Joan and I would follow. Cancer was a secret in my childhood family. No one was supposed to know. My mother died believing—I am certain falsely—that my father (a 200-pound man who dwindled to 100 pounds) did not know he had cancer. My brother, Steve, only learned of it a few months before our father's death. I learned my father had died of cancer when Steve gently broke the news of his death as I was being driven back from my summer camp on August 4, 1959, to attend his funeral.

Notwithstanding these differences of style, years later Joan and I would reflect on how much I learned from my mother about giving care.

And the experience of not knowing that my father was dying, not being able to say good-bye, left scars that Joan and I hope we have addressed in how we handled her illness with our children.

From fifth grade through high school, I attended the Riverdale Country School. For the first few years, I lived in the dormitory, a cause of much loneliness but also a means of protecting me from the sadness and turmoil in my family. There were other important sources of support. Elvie Lorig, a refugee from Nazi Germany, was our "second mother," providing Steve and me with love and structure—even into the present. My aunt Gloria and uncle Bill Meyers, Nora Campbell, teachers, and close friends were also supportive.

A kind kid and a good athlete, I was "spaced out" and a mediocre student. I was devastated by my father's death. I still recall the feeling I had in my stomach, an aching that something had been torn away, leaving a hole that could never be filled.

Graduating with a less than stellar academic record, I attended Boston University where I did fairly well and found much of my life's direction through involvement in the civil rights and antiwar movements. After college, I held several community service positions, traveled around the United States, built potter's kick wheels, ran a political campaign . . . No great accomplishments, simply an often unhappy young adult trying to find himself in life, work, and love. A master's degree in public administration at Northeastern University was followed by doctoral studies at Brandeis University. At Brandeis I found my professional direction. More important, I found Joan during this period.

CANINE INTRODUCTIONS: 1977–1979

Joan and I were introduced by our dogs, Leda and Solo, in the late summer of 1977. I was walking, and she was running, in a park off of Route 117 in Lincoln, Massachusetts. After talking a bit about our dogs, I encouraged her to stop by after her run, telling her where I was going to be. Disappointed that she did not stop by my reading spot, I returned to the car to find a note on the windshield that said "Sorry, got stung by a bee.

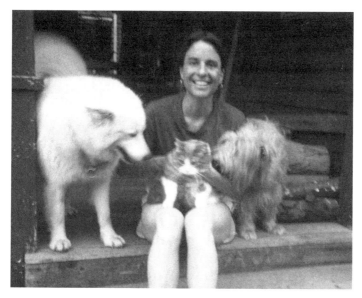

Canine introductions: Leda, Joan, Francis the cat, and Solo, 1977.

Had to go home." The note was written on the back of an envelope addressed to her. Subtle and effective. I saved the note and made plans to call her.

I can't say that I had a feeling that I had met my future wife, but I recall telling a Jewish friend that he would be pleased to know that I finally met a "nice Jewish girl." At least I thought I had, because Joan "looked Jewish." More important, I was correct about her being nice.

A couple of months passed and we began to date, deciding within a year to live together with Solo and Leda and Francis, the cat. As I neared the completion of my dissertation and the beginning of an academic career, Joan made it clear that we needed to make a decision about our future. Living with me in the Boston area was one thing, but picking up and moving to another city required more of a commitment—marriage. Did I want to make such a commitment? Could I maintain this commitment? I could be monogamous for awhile, but for life! Would marriage be a straitjacket? I thought about life with and life without Joan. With and without children. With and without the grounding that marriage implies. I arranged for a dozen red roses to be delivered to Joan while dining at the Concord Inn. The note read, "Will you marry me?" "Yes," thank God, the response. We committed to each other and we kept that commitment.

We were married on April 29, 1979, by a rabbi and a priest, with friends and family present. At the beginning of the ceremony, the rabbi announced that—for the "benefit of the Jews in the audience"—he would be sure to immediately translate any Hebrew he used into English.

WE MOVE TO BALTIMORE

We moved to Baltimore that August, where I had accepted a position as an assistant professor at the University of Maryland's School of Social Work and where Joan would find work in various child development roles, primarily with hospitalized children. The first couple of years were very difficult—too many changes, too little confidence, and too much anxiety. My first teaching experiences terrified me. First couple of classes, I prayed that I would not faint dead away in the classroom. Each class felt like an exam. I worked constantly, writing articles when I was not preparing for class. Joan took over a classroom of twelve acting-out, emotionally disturbed children that the Baltimore school system deemed unsuitable for inclusion in the city's special education programs. Coming home exhausted and sometimes bruised, she blamed herself for having so much difficulty with the assignment. No one provided supervision or feedback to her. Only after leaving the job did she learn that she was valued (as she always was) as an outstanding teacher, and that she had managed to stay with this classroom longer and more effectively than any of her predecessors.

We were both highly anxious and depressed. Awaking early one morning, I turned toward Joan and commented on how nervous I felt, how unhappy I was. This precipitated our marriage's only incident of "family violence." Smacking me with her fist three times in the middle of my chest, Joan said, "I hate the University of Maryland, I hate the

Children's Guild, I hate Baltimore. I want to go home to Boston." We cried and then went to work.

Fortunately, we didn't pick up stakes. Life went on and we calmed down. With time I learned to tolerate my work, and with more time to greatly value teaching. I became more settled in my role as an academic, finding time to conduct research and write. Joan found a position she enjoyed in the Child Life Department of Johns Hopkins Hospital, working with children with cancer and training students to work in child development roles with hospitalized children.

Hearing about Joan's kids and their families, I often wondered how they did it. Where did these children find the strength? How could their parents bear the pain of having a child with cancer? How could the family travel weekly from all over for treatment? How could many of the families maintain humor and love of life? How could the parents care for a sick child, their other children, and hold paid employment? How could people find such strength; be so exceptional? As Joan said then (and as we later learned), families do what they have to do. Faced with serious illness of this sort, you really do not have a lot of choices. If you are "fortunate" to find the strength within (and I believe many individuals and families are), you just "do it." What looks like heroism to others is often something these families have no control over. They simply could not do it any other way.

ADIRONDACK SUMMERS

During these early years in Baltimore, we began taking our summer vacations in the Adirondacks. We only missed two of these "Adirondack summers"—1982, when Aaron was born, and 1992, when the family was in Australia. For the first ten years, we rented different cottages near Lake Champlain in Essex, New York. Having established a summer tradition that we, and later our children, loved, we purchased a farmhouse a few miles north in Willsboro, New York, in 1989. A terrible financial decision, it turned into a wonderful investment in our family and friends.

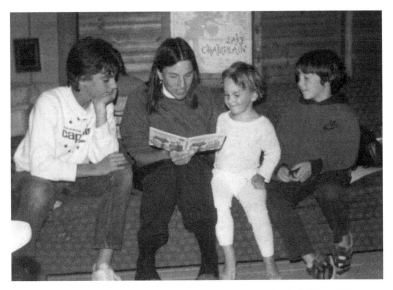

Joan reading to Aaron and her nephews, Anders Fernbach (left) and Peter Fernbach (right), 1986.

Our professions allowed us to spend sometimes as many as six weeks in upstate New York. Over the years, the cottage rentals and later our Willsboro home became a source of connection—to each other, our children, family, and friends. While I often worked during these vacations, especially during the early years, there was plenty of time to slow down. Long walks, campfires, fishing, canoeing, meals, swimming holes, lakes, an occasional camping trip, and visits from our families and close friends occupied our time. In Willsboro, Joan was often busy in the yard and I with household repairs.

The Adirondacks are a place of birth and renewal for Joan and me. We made decisions to become parents there. Later, our summer home became a place of sustenance. After diagnosis, we managed to have two summers there, not as carefree as we had hoped but still wonderful. It is in the Adirondacks, more than anywhere else, that Joan imagined her spirit would rest, waiting by campfires for each of us to come in turn. And it was in Willsboro, shortly after she died, that during a waking moment I caught my first glimpse of Joan smiling as if to say, "hurry up, Eric, there's work to be done."

OUR FAMILY GROWS

Well, back to Baltimore. Our lives were good, much better than we may have realized. We enjoyed living in a small village-like area on the edge of the city. New friendships developed. We, especially Joan, seemed to have a knack for developing warm relationships with our neighbors. Our immediate neighbors, Charles and Georgine Sumwalt, later became "god-grandparents" to our children. We shared many afternoon talks and weekend crab feasts on their back porch. One day I returned home to find Charles, then about seventy-six years old, on our roof fixing our chimney. Joan maintained an especially close, even somewhat flirtatious, relationship with Charles right up until her death.

Joan walked Solo and Leda at least twice a day by the stream that ran through the center of this small community, developing many acquaintances and a lasting friendship with Michele Melville, who was present when Joan died. Liela Amsel, a friend who lived near the stream, suffered from adult-onset cystic fibrosis. Joan would stop by Liela's nearly every day and they would take walks or later, as Liela's condition deteriorated, just sit. Liela, a fighter, would not give up, even as each breath became increasingly more labored. When Liela's time to die came, Joan was saddened by how she suffered. More pain medication was needed, and even Liela's husband, a caring physician, had difficulty gaining access to the necessary narcotic agents. It was the early 1980s, and pain management techniques were more limited than they are today. But more than Liela's suffering, her strength in the face of a critical illness made a permanent impression on Joan.

Taking a leave of absence from the University of Maryland, I commuted to Washington during 1982 to serve as an adviser to the 1982–1993 National Commission on Social Security Reform. This was a period of tremendous professional growth. But for us, Aaron's birth was the big event of 1982.

Joan was not dogmatic about natural childbirth or breast-feeding or later about how to die, though she had clear preferences. Twenty plus hours into labor, she agreed to use Pitocin to "hasten" Aaron's delivery, and he made his debut calmly a few hours later. When Aaron did not gain weight, Joan, very worried and feeling like she was failing as a mother, agreed at first suggestion to supplement her breast-feeding with formula. Aaron did well.

Joan and I were absolutely thrilled at being parents. Aaron was an "easy" and pensive baby, and later toddler. As he grew, I built a playhouse and sandbox; Joan made these structures come alive through patient play with him and later Johanna. We didn't have family supports nearby. Michele, whose first child Sarah was then three years old, became an especially close friend and guide to Joan throughout early motherhood. Howie Baum, who worked with me at the university, and his wife Madelyn Siegel, a psychiatrist with an oncology background, rejoiced in the growth of our family, even as they struggled to have their own children. Later, when they adopted Elena and Maya, we were able to return this warmth.

Joan was as wonderful and caring a mother as there is. If anything, she was too caring, often sacrificing her needs for the family's—an occasional source of marital tensions. (Not a bad indictment of a spouse to say she gave too much to her children, her husband, and to her dogs and cats!) A proud and doting father, I had much to learn about being fully attentive to our children, about giving baths, and later about listening. I was certainly "there," but I was also busy with professional advancement and earning a few extra dollars. Joan spent six months at home with Aaron and then returned to her work at Johns Hopkins. The Social Security commission issued its report and I returned to the University of Maryland.

Life continued. I worried about getting tenure. Joan worried about the children at Hopkins. Believing in the importance of creating opportunities for hospitalized children to express themselves through play and social interaction, she sometimes expressed frustration at the status afforded to child life specialists in medical settings. Her work was important to children and their families, but I'll confess to believing that it was an uphill battle for it to gain the respect it deserved by other medical professionals.

Two Adirondack summers passed, the second leading to Johanna's conception in our rented cottage.

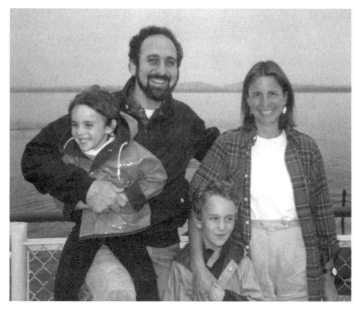

Johanna, Eric, Aaron, and Joan, Adirondack summer, 1988.

Johanna, born quickly and with a flair in May 1985, was active from the "git-go"—the one baby in constant motion in the hospital's nursery. More than once during Johanna's infancy, a stranger stopped Joan to say with a knowing smile, "I had one like this. She never stopped being active."

Our day-to-day lives became more split—hers on home and mine on work. Joan, fond of saying that it is not true that "you can have it all," cut back to part-time work—sacrificing career advancement for family. Frustrated with the academic environment and seeking a little extra income, I took another leave of absence when given the opportunity to direct a study of emerging issues in aging for the Gerontological Society of America—again commuting to Washington.

I was offered a new position at Boston College's Graduate School of Social Work along with a promotion to associate professor. It seemed unlikely that I would be offered tenure at Maryland, and my salary was quite low. We agreed that it made sense to move while the kids were still young, four and one. But Joan was very sad. She loved our home and she had—as she always would—made it a real home. I liked our home, but I worried that our quaint 150-year-old farmhouse might fall apart before we could afford necessary repairs. She liked our neighbors and community. I did too, but felt we needed to move because there was too much crime and the public schools were not adequate. Where Joan saw mostly loss, I saw mostly opportunity. Also, we had many good friends and family in the Boston area, including Joan's sisters, Catherine and Mary Jo.

CREATING A NEW HOME IN NATICK

I accepted the position. We sold our house in the flat Baltimore housing market. We packed our Baltimore home into a rental van and I drove it to our new house in Natick, Massachusetts, stopping only in New York City to pick up my lifelong friend George Igel. George offered to keep me company on the drive and probably thought I would need his skills as a psychiatrist as I pondered our new mortgage and dealt with the guilt of wrenching Joan from our Baltimore home. This was to be our last move because, as Joan said, she couldn't go through the pain of doing this again.

Within a couple of years we were comfortably settled in Natick, involved in the kids' schools, later in soccer, and, once again, getting to know our neighbors. Life was good; again, better than I realized. Our new house lacked the charm of our Baltimore home, but with time it became even more of a home. Joan cultivated the yard and flowers. I wanted to have another child but recognized that this was not my call. Joan said, as she often did when wanting to avoid conflict, "Let's see." We got a new puppy, and as we drove her home the quiet realization came on me that the dog was as close to a third child as we would get. Johanna, who had few memories of her time in Baltimore but knew from whence she had come, immediately suggested we name the puppy "Baltimore." It stuck.

Joan took Baltimore on daily morning and evening walks and often on two- to three-mile runs. I began coaching Aaron's soccer teams. As

Johanna came of soccer age, Joan joined me in coaching her teams. I lost thirty pounds (something I need to do again!) and started playing in over-thirty and later over-forty and over-fifty men's soccer leagues. Christmases, Hanukkahs, Passovers, Easters, and Thanksgivings came and went, marked by family celebrations. Natick was now home. And, as a note I recently received from Johanna's childhood friend Deirdre Salsich reminds, our home was warm and open to our children's friends. Deirdre wrote:

> I've been thinking about you, Aaron, and Johanna a lot lately as the anniversary of Joan's death approaches. I continue to think of her often. She was such an influential person in my life. Some of my fondest childhood memories are of intramural soccer with you and Joan. You both made me and every other kid you coached think that they could do anything. Your home was always a warm, welcoming place. I feel like I did a lot of growing up on Sawin Street and in the Adirondacks. Your family has given me so much strength and guidance throughout my life, and I am so grateful. Whenever I feel proud of a paper, a race, or anything I've achieved, I feel as though Joan has had a hand in it somehow. She was such an inspirational person for so many, and I feel her presence in the kindred friends I hold so dear.
>
> May this letter find you rested and surrounded by family and friends.

Joan and I had an ambivalent relationship with religion. Neither of us felt comfortable with religious institutions, at least not in the way we experienced them in childhood. We both often felt the presence of God, of a spirit, in our lives—especially during quiet times on walks or with our family. Joan liked some of the rituals of the Catholic Church but rejected what she considered its rigidities. I have a strong identity of myself as a Jew but rejected the materialism of temples I was exposed to as a child. Also, being Hebrew-impaired, I always found my mind wandering to other places in temple.

Teaching at a Catholic university, living in an area of Natick that was largely Catholic and not having Jewish family close by, I was concerned that our children be exposed to their Jewish heritage, but it took a while for Joan and me to really address this. Once we talked about it, I realized that Joan was comfortable with raising the kids in a loose Jewish manner as long as I would take the lead. We affiliated with a couple of Jewish groups that celebrated holidays together. The kids didn't resonate with the Sunday school, so we made different, and what turned out to be more effective, arrangements (at least for us). We asked Evelyn Melacon, a former teacher at the school and a friend, if she would meet with Aaron, and later Johanna, to prepare them for their bar and bat mitzvahs. Of course, probably to Evelyn's chagrin, we still celebrated Christmas and Easter and only lit the Sabbath lights, if the truth be known, maybe once a month.

We held two very special celebrations of the kid's journeys toward adulthood. Evelyn's two sons, Jake and Dan, joined Aaron in bar mitzvah in 1995. Johanna's 1998 bat mitzvah also brought together our many friends just before we moved to Syracuse. Held in our backyard under a large tent, Evelyn presided over the services with participation by other family and friends. While lacking a rabbi and an excess of Hebrew, God could only be pleased by the warmth and pleasure that was given expression in both events. In my, and I believe many other people's experiences, only Joan's funeral held in a tent in the backyard of our Syracuse home three years after Johanna's bat mitzvah, carried a greater sense of emotion and connection among those present.

Again, years passed and several themes wove through our lives—continued joy in our children, pleasure in being part of a community, tensions related to dissatisfactions we both had in our work, and a maturing of our relationship that did not come without some strains.

Joan was teaching at Wheelock College, directing a graduate program that trained students for child life positions, primarily in hospital settings. A terrific teacher, competent administrator, and clear writer, Joan had all the skills to do very well in an academic environment. But she didn't have a PhD, and she wasn't particularly interested in getting

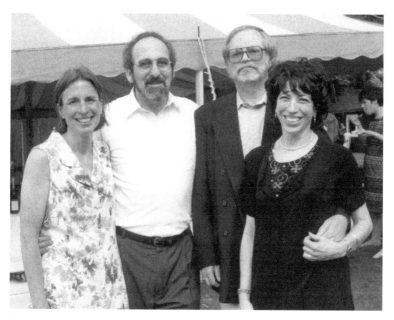

Joan, Eric, and Scott and Susan Plumb celebrate Johanna's bat mitzvah,
1998. Courtesy of Judy Salsich.

one. In some ways this was a setup. She liked the flexibility of academic
work, the creativity it sometimes encourages, and working with child
life students. She disliked the self-righteousness and status consciousness that often drives academic politics. Her students valued her teaching, and many stayed in contact after graduating as had some families
that Joan worked with at Hopkins. After a few years, Joan was asked to
apply for a tenure-track position at Wheelock. One of the few people in
academic life who did not want a permanent tenured position, she ap-
plied because she had no other alternative if she wanted to stay at
Wheelock. She was hired (they would have been crazy not to hire her.)

Joan could be very intense, even anxious about her work. She had
colleagues and friends on the faculty, like Marcia Hartley, who became
something of a cross between an older sister and a mother to Joan, as
well as Muriel Hirt, Stefi Rubin, Dick Thompson, and others. But Joan
didn't respect how some people treated each other at Wheelock. Even

so, she needed some professional pats on the back from some of these same people and was frustrated and at times angry when her own and other colleagues' good work was not acknowledged. Without a PhD, she felt (and was) treated by some faculty as a second-rate citizen. But, still, she had no interest in entering doctoral studies.

Instead, she decided to get a nursing degree. She began taking the requisite chemistry and biology courses to enter a nursing program. Although accepted in a nurse-practitioner program, she decided on a BSN program at Boston College. She took a partial, then a full leave of absence from Wheelock College. She was excited by the prospect of learning a concrete set of skills that would allow her to combine her interests in child development and health education. I think she realized a few months into the program full time that she may have made the wrong choice. But Joan was committed, and once committed she was exceptionally determined to do very well.

I never saw anyone work so hard (except possibly our daughter!). During this period (1995 to 1998), Joan did not have much time for herself. She did not compromise the kids or me. She remained the center of home. She was up early and late doing her course work. The kids saw a mother who was a serious and outstanding student, not an insignificant model for their pre-college years. The "oldest" nursing undergrad, Joan was liked and respected by students and faculty. She recognized that some of the teaching was poor and some of the assignments little more than busywork. She was offended, not much for herself but for the young students who were being put through the nursing education process, by the rigidity and at times near sadism exhibited by a few nursing instructors. Despite this, she wanted to excel. And, even with her maturity and her understanding of the weaknesses in the program, it stung when she received a grade less than an "A." I remember her crying when a teacher she knew had it in for her gave her a B+! A few years later as she dealt with her cancer, we laughed at what a waste of energy it was to be troubled by this. But I suspect it still bothered her.

Meanwhile, my career continued to unfold at Boston College. Superficially, you could say I was doing well. I was tenured after three years. I continued to receive the type of recognition that marks a successful academic career. The teaching was mostly fun. I liked my students. Boston College had many good resources and there were people outside my department, and some within, whom I liked and respected. But the departmental environment was poisonous. Over my twelve years at the Graduate School of Social Work, more often than not, I saw many good and honest people—faculty, staff, and students—be mistreated, be defined as "problematic," lose their employment, fail to receive tenure, and so forth. Where I show respect by stating my views forthrightly and feel a professional obligation to do so, the culture and leadership of the school interpreted honest disagreement as an affront. Compliant and self-centered people who did not question the administrative direction of the school, even if a student or colleague was being unfairly harmed, tended to thrive. I was angered at the nastiness and too reactive. I became increasingly unhappy, depressed at times. The only Jew ever tenured at the Boston College Graduate School of Social Work since its founding in 1936, I was reminded more than once by the school's dean that I was a first. This said, the unpleasantness I experienced had relatively little to do with anti-Semitism. I simply could not accept the way the school was run and did not respect its leadership or those who sat by silently.

But we liked living in Natick and there were other incentives to stay, including many positives at Boston College. Besides, I was always hoping that the administrative structure of the school might turn over. (It did. Two years after I left!)

As relations at the school deteriorated, I focused on my writing and teaching and began looking forward to a 1993 sabbatical. The sabbatical year came and we were able to take the kids out of the country for four months. Another terrible financial decision, but one of the best things we did. We spent two weeks in New Zealand, where Joan facilitated a conference on child life education for the first week. I spent three months as a visiting scholar at the University of Queensland in Brisbane, Australia. Aaron went to school for some of this time and Joan made various attempts to home school Johanna without killing her. I earned my stripes as an assistant coach for Aaron's "Tarringa Soccer Club" team. I had a good experience at the university and learned about the Australian income security system. Fortunately we took some time to play, visiting Melbourne, Sydney, Canberra, and some of Queensland's more remote areas. The highlight of the trip was three weeks spent in Fiji, providing all of us with the opportunity to experience a very different culture.

The trip was worth every penny and more. It was a good family experience, a source of stories that continue to this day, and an "adventure" that heightened our family's connections to each other. After returning home, Aaron, asked to find Boston on a globe, pointed to Australia and said, "Here's Australia. Now you go up and over and down and here's Boston." Our understandings of the world and even each other had

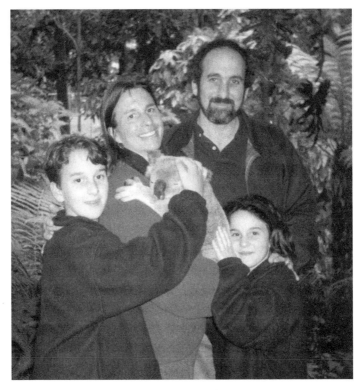

Aaron, Joan, Eric, and Johanna in Australia, 1993.

changed. More than once, during the years that Joan dealt with cancer, each of us said how fortunate we were to take this time together.

Returning to Boston College in the fall of 1993, things went from bad to worse. I managed my spirits on a day-to-day basis by laughing and venting with several colleagues and tennis buddies. Soccer—coaching and playing—provided an increasingly important outlet. Family life remained good, but it was not without tensions—much related to my unhappiness at work. An opportunity came along in 1994 that allowed me to take a six-month leave of absence to serve as a senior adviser to another presidential commission, the Bipartisan Commission on Entitlement and Tax Reform. I commuted to Washington, again hoping that my leave might coincide with administrative turnover. No such luck. Throughout much of this time, Joan wondered whether I could just make peace and stop tilting at windmills.

Returning once again to the faculty, the environment was even worse. My closest colleague and faculty friend, Paul Wilson, was now the target of the dean and her colleagues. Paul made the "mistake" of not turning his back on mistreated colleagues or students, of quietly and thoughtfully offering his views. Paul's fall from grace may have begun a few years earlier when he supported the appeal of an assistant professor who a university committee later determined was unfairly denied tenure. The dean, in spite of strong efforts by a couple of us, terminated Paul's contract in 1996. Without warning, the associate dean delivered the message late in the academic year: Paul's contract would not be renewed. Joan was appalled. She had the highest regard for Paul as a calm and competent person with much integrity. Combined with some of her experiences with the rigidities of Boston College's School of Nursing, she was now more sympathetic to the difficulties I was having at the school.

Joan continued to make progress toward her nursing degree, including starting her clinical training at Beth Israel and other settings. She had great respect for nursing before her clinicals and even more once she had firsthand experience with how much needed to be done for the few patients in her care. I published another book or two and continued to coach and play soccer. We redid our kitchen in Natick. Holidays continued to come and go. We were frustrated with the quality of education being offered in our children's middle school, but continued to greatly value the experience of raising children in the context of the neighborhood and larger community.

Walking back from a tennis game and talking about my problems at the school, my friend John Williamson said something like, "You never know; these may be the good old days." I've thought about this comment many times after moving to Syracuse. John didn't mean it this way, but he was right. The problems I had at BC seem so small now. But how was I to know this then?

My commitment to staying in the Boston area continued to erode. With Joan's agreement, during the spring of 1997 I explored the possibility of applying for a position at Syracuse University's School of Social Work. I liked what I saw, especially the friendliness and openness of the faculty. Joan gave me the go-ahead to apply, and I was offered a tenured full professorship. I was ready, but we were not. Joan was willing, but not pleased, to move. Aaron was accepting and Johanna didn't like the

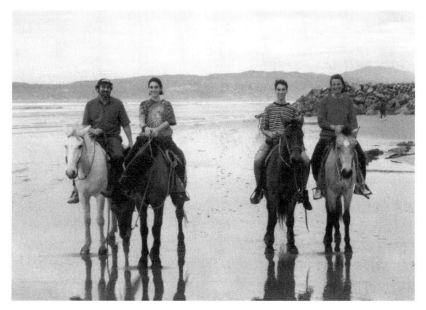

Eric, Johanna, Aaron, and Joan, family vacation in Mexico, Christmas 1997.

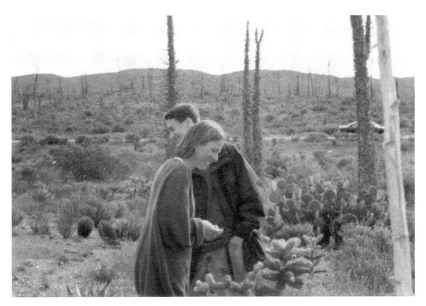

Joan and Aaron laughing after Dad backed into some cactus! 1997.

idea at all. As we explored the move further, I realized that Joan would have a very difficult time finishing her degree and that she most likely would not. But, probably more than anything else, a tragedy in our neighborhood figured into our decision to turn the job down. A nineteen-year-old boy who was one of our first Natick babysitters committed suicide. The neighborhood was devastated. In this grief we were reminded of how connected we were to the community. I turned the job down, fully intending to remain in Natick.

The next year, however, after my promotion to full professor was undermined by my dean, Joan and I decided that enough was enough. It was sad contemplating leaving. I reapplied for the Syracuse position. Joan completed her work on her nursing degree. I was offered the job. I considered trying to negotiate a position for Joan at Syracuse University. Joan, after all, was giving up a tenure-track position at Wheelock College. Characteristically, she said not to muddy the waters, believing she would find worthwhile work once she got the family settled. Indeed, she did, but not the type she imagined.

In May, Joan graduated magna cum laude with a near perfect (3.96) GPA, of which I remain very proud, even though I wish she had spent her time in a more pleasant way. On the day of her graduation, Joan, Aaron, Johanna, and I celebrated with a late lunch at the Concord Inn, the same restaurant where years earlier I had proposed and where we had our pre-wedding family dinner. She was feeling under the weather with a stomachache, one that lasted most of the day. She chalked it up to anxiety over all the changes coming our way.

I accepted the position at Syracuse University. We placed our house on the market. Johanna's bat mitzvah brought most of our friends and neighbors together one more time at our Natick home. Seeing them and Johanna's friends, some of whom we had coached for several years, we were again reminded of how much we valued our years there and how much we would leave behind. Moving day came and went in early July. We spent a week setting up our new home in Manlius, New York, and then went to the Adirondacks to relax for several weeks before our new adventure was to begin.

At the time, my worst fear was that Joan would be lonely and that her job search would get her down. How I wish that had been the case . . .

3

Diagnosis

FROM HEMORRHOIDS TO CANCER

☙ Joan likened the period of diagnosis to going to a movie where one tragedy after another befalls the main characters. As she put it, "You cry your eyes out and then go home saying, 'Thank God, it was only a movie.' The trouble is, it's not!"

Initial diagnosis and then deciding what to do about the cancer were two of the most difficult periods in our thirty-two-month marathon. The information we received during this six-week period changed our lives. Forever. We were "crazed." But we also managed, with George Igel's and other people's advice, to carefully explore treatment options and to make good choices about physicians and treatments.

Dealing with cancer has been likened to riding a roller coaster—lots of ups and downs and unexpected twists. As we started our ride, we were in steep fall. Each test, each piece of information, was progressively more discouraging than the last. By mid-October 1998, we had been told that Joan had advanced colon cancer that had metastasized to the liver. We wryly joked that we were waiting for some "ups."

EARLY WARNINGS: A BOTCHED COLONOSCOPY

Joan turned forty-seven on September 1, 1998, six weeks prior to her diagnosis. With the exception of the stomachaches that had increased in frequency during the summer, Joan seemed to be in excellent health. She

35

exercised regularly, often running or walking a few miles each day. She ate well, very little red meat and lots of vegetables, especially broccoli! She could have served as a poster child for a healthy lifestyle.

The cancer should have been diagnosed nine months earlier. If it had been, perhaps she would still be here.

Joan caught the commuter train to Boston early on January 21, 1998. She was in the final semester of her nursing degree and on the way to her nursing practicum.

I received an unexpected call shortly after she arrived at Boston's South Station. She was very worried. She had just had a frightening rectal bleed. At the risk of being indelicate, I'll simply say that she observed that the blood was embedded in the stool, not floating around as is usually the case with hemorrhoidal bleeds. And there was a fair amount of blood.

After talking, she called our HMO, Harvard-Vanguard, and arranged for an evening appointment. Expressing concern at the amount of bleeding, the on-call doc arranged for a colonoscopy the following morning. He considered hospitalizing her that night but felt it safe to discharge her as long as she would monitor the bleeding and call the emergency number if needed. She prepped for the test. We went to sleep.

We showed up bright and early at the endoscopy center of a major Boston hospital. Joan wasn't looking forward to the procedure, and she was clearly worried about what the test might show. She went into the treatment area. I waited. She came back and told me the test was horrible, but that she had been told by the doctor that she was fine. Hemorrhoids. Nothing else.

Walking outside the hospital, she told me the test had been extremely painful. Now here I have to confess to being a bit inattentive. I heard Joan explain how the nurses had trouble putting the IV in her and how the anesthesia (Fentanyl and Versed) was only running a few minutes prior to the start of the procedure. I heard her say that the doctor said that people with tight stomach muscles (that is, runners) sometimes have a harder time with the procedure (an opinion no other docs have corroborated). I heard her say that the procedure was more painful than the natural deliveries of Aaron and Johanna. But I was simply relieved. A diagnosis of hemorrhoids and a few minutes of pain beat a pain-free diagnosis of cancer. The pain was transitory. We could go about our daily lives.

Nine months would pass before we would learn that the procedure had not been completed; that the doctor stopped short of examining the entire colon. Reading through Joan's Harvard-Vanguard medical record, we came across the following: "Videocolonoscopy performed to 100 cm, at which point the patient had pain and despite multiple positioning, we could go no further. Got to about transverse colon, possibly as far as the hepatic flexure. Entire colon well seen, no polyps or growths. There were internal hemorrhoids."

Unfortunately, Joan's tumor was in the area that was not visualized, in the cecum, the area just before the juncture where the colon joins the small intestines. Had the doctor completed the test, there is no way the tumor could have been missed. But it was. So, we went off pleased that everything was fine.

Would Joan have gone back for another colonoscopy if she had been told the procedure wasn't completed? Absolutely. She was careful with her health. But there was no reason for Joan or her regular health care providers to challenge a diagnosis of hemorrhoids. She had been tested and she was fine. And we were all invested in her remaining so.

So, in May, when Joan had a stomachache on her day of graduation from Boston College, it was natural for her to chalk it up to stress. We had a bat mitzvah planned for a week later, our house was on the market, and we were getting ready to move. Besides, she had already been tested. And when she had another stomachache in late June, we were in the midst of our move. And . . .

It was not until early August, while on our vacation in the Adirondacks, that we began to worry and that Joan voiced her fear that something was not right. In mid-August, I asked Joan about going to Burlington, Vermont, to see a doctor. She thought it made sense to wait until we got back to Syracuse in a couple of weeks. We waited.

THE LABOR DAY TORNADO

Our return home was marked by a tornado, a minor inconvenience compared to what was to follow.

During Labor Day weekend, tornado-level winds plunged Syracuse, and much of central New York, into a state of emergency. Sunday night we awoke to almost constant lightning and high winds. A few minutes later, Johanna came into our bed scared. As the winds literally shook the walls of our house, she calmly suggested we go to the basement. Good idea. (Why didn't I think of that!) Bruised ego notwithstanding, we quickly followed her advice, awakening Aaron, bringing blankets, radio and flashlights, and, of course, our dog Baltimore and Billie the cat.

Emerging a few hours later, we were relieved to find that we still had a house. There was damage—lost trees, broken windows, water, strained attic beams, no electricity—but nothing that would prevent us from living in our home. Our neighbors, the Luxes, weren't so fortunate. Their roofing was strewn over their neighbors' yards.

In the days that followed, we began the cleanup, arranging for repairs and documenting the damage for our insurance company. We and much of the region were without electricity for almost a week. My classes at Syracuse University were disrupted. This was certainly not how we had expected to begin our residence in Syracuse. Little did we know!

INITIAL DIAGNOSIS

Diagnosis began innocently enough. Joan's first Syracuse appointment on September 3 was with Deborah Schu, the nurse-practitioner who would guide her through diagnosis and connect us with outstanding health care providers. Knowing that Joan wanted to avoid another colonoscopy, and suspecting it would not be needed, Debbie arranged for a CT scan for the next day.

The CT results did not seem terribly worrisome. "The liver, spleen, pancreas, adrenal glands and kidneys are unremarkable," the report told us. There was some "apparent thickening of the ascending colon and cecal region," possibly "related to incomplete distension rather than a true abnormality." A barium enema was suggested to rule out "the possibility of a mass."

Interpretation of medical lingo: The smart money was on Joan having an uncomfortable, but far from life-threatening, condition such as diverticulitis or irritable bowel syndrome.

But, as suggested, she took the next step toward diagnosis, still relieved that no one had suggested another colonoscopy.

The barium enema results were worrisome, more than we recognized at the time. The September 16 report noted the "possibility of a sessile mass" in the area of the cecum and recommended a follow-up endoscopic procedure. Another step toward being redefined as a family dealing with cancer.

Joan was worried, less so about the possible "sessile mass" than about the increasingly frequent abdominal pains she was having and the need to go through another colonoscopic procedure. The first one had been so painful. Debbie referred Joan to Dr. Mark Kasowitz, a gastroenterologist.

We met with Dr. Kasowitz. Joan was clear. She just wanted to be knocked out, to not experience the pain she had in Boston. Dr. Kasowitz promised to use lots of Versed and Fentanyl. The appointment was set for September 24.

We still were not all that worried. Expectations of an irritable bowel or diverticulitis diagnosis kept our anxiety relatively low. Besides, Joan was too healthy to have cancer.

Dr. Kasowitz kept his promise. Joan was made comfortable and drifted off. I left to teach an hour-long class, expecting everything to be fine. Halfway into my class, I was called out and told that I should call Dr. Kasowitz. I borrowed a cell phone from a student and called. Dr. Kasowitz got on the line saying that I should come over to his office to be present when Joan awakened. "How bad is the news?" There was a good-sized tumor. "Shit! Pardon my reaction, but . . ." I thought about my father dying from colon cancer. This couldn't happen again.

Fifteen minutes later, I was by Joan in the recovery area. She was still sedated and unaware of what was unfolding. As her eyes opened, Dr. Kasowitz came by her bed and began to explain that he found two polyps, one too large to take out during the colonoscopy. He had taken several biopsies. "How worried should we be?" In his experience, this type of polyp presented as if it was cancerous. But if it were, it could probably be handled surgically, since it didn't appear that the tumor had broken through the wall of the colon.

The biopsy results came back negative. We were relieved, but Dr. Kasowitz warned that he still thought it could be cancerous.

He recommended a consult with Dr. Dennis Brown. We were assured by several medical practitioners that Dr. Brown was very capable, the type of doctor that doctors would choose for themselves. Even so, we sent the various diagnostic reports and films to our former physician at Harvard-Vanguard in Massachusetts. Is surgery necessary, we asked. Yes. Is a general surgeon appropriate for this surgery? Yes. We spoke with several friends who are physicians. They agreed that surgery was the way to go. Nothing fancy about this. Just get it over with.

We met with Dr. Brown. We liked him immediately. He had a calm and reassuring demeanor. He reminded us of Joan's brother, Dennis. He addressed Joan as "Joanie," an endearment that only Dennis, her father, and a couple of family members ever used. He was patient with our questions. "Were we dealing with cancer?" He didn't know, but if it were, he did not expect it to be invasive.

Dr. Brown took time to explain the surgery he proposed—a resection of the colon. It was like splicing a hose. The part of the colon that had the tumors would be snipped and then the colon would be reconnected. A pretty standard procedure to a surgeon, but he understood it was anything but standard to us.

We asked about laparoscopic surgery. We had learned that this technique was now being used to excise abdominal tumors. He was open to our exploring this option, but he did not think it was advisable given the size of the tumor—4 to 5 centimeters. Yes, it would allow for quicker and more comfortable recovery, but there was greater danger of spreading cells if the tumor was cancerous. We asked him about the anesthesia.

Yes, the anesthesiologist would be present. Yes, he would take special precautions, knowing that Joan had once had a difficult time with anesthesia during an earlier surgery.

We set a date: Tuesday, October 6, 1998.

The abdominal pains had become more frequent and more intense. Joan was ready for the surgery. She just wanted to get rid of the pain and get on with her life. I was nervous. I had lost my mother in a surgery that was less invasive. I worried that Joan might not come out of the anesthesia. To pass time, we busied ourselves fixing up our home. The weekend before her surgery, I changed most of the electrical switches in our home—my way of trying to fix everything.

SURGERY

The morning of the surgery went well. Dr. Brown was calm and reassuring. An IV drip was started. Joan was wheeled into the OR, and I retired to the waiting room. Alejandro Garcia, my friend and colleague at Syracuse University, joined me as soon as his class was over. We waited. I worried. We waited.

Dr. Brown appeared after a couple of hours. The surgery was over, and Joan had done well. She was coming out of the anesthesia and would be brought to her room in an hour or so.

"I know you cannot be certain and I know it's not fair to ask, but what is your impression of the tumor? Just your instinct, Dr. Brown."

"I think Joanie is going to be fine, but we'll know for sure when we get the report from pathology." He mentioned that the tumor felt like it was benign. And it seemed well encapsulated.

"Thank God. And thank you, Dr. Brown." Alejandro hugged me.

A little later, Joan was brought to her room. We were relieved. The surgery had gone well. The exhaustion and postsurgical pain would pass. I connected to the Internet with my portable computer and sent out an e-mail to family and friends saying it looked as if we were out of the woods. I spread out sheets and pillows on a recliner and managed to get some sleep between beeps and blood pressure checks.

Early in the morning, a tall, pleasant Haitian woman awakened Joan, coaxing her with warm humor to take a short walk. Yes, they really do get you up and moving as quickly as possible after abdominal surgery! Walking helps get the insides working again and helps to prevent scar tissue from building up.

Joan got up slowly, very slowly, and very hunched, straightening herself out as much she could. The tubing was draped over the IV pole, and off she went for the longest sixty yards of her life. The nurse's aide supported her, and I pushed the IV pole, watching that she not get entangled. She returned to bed exhausted.

The day went on. By evening, we had taken several walks through the halls, including one six-lap walk—about half a mile, we figured. The nurses and aids smiled as Joan made her rounds. Friendly quips were exchanged as patients passed each other in the hall. Things were pretty upbeat. Looked as if we had dodged this bullet.

Night came. Ever practical, and always concerned about the kids, Joan sent me packing. "I'm doing okay, Eric. You go home and see the kids. And get a good night's sleep."

At home, I checked in with Aaron and Johanna. I don't really remember the evening, but it was the last that cancer would not be a central fact of our lives.

NO NEWS WAS GOOD NEWS

On the morning of Thursday, October 8, 1998, the telephone rang. It was Joan, and the news was not good. Dr. Brown had stopped by Joan's room earlier than expected. The pathology was back. The tumor tested positive for cancer, including some lymph nodes. That's all I could hear. Joan had cancer. She was scared and I was scared.

"I love you, sweetheart. We'll figure this out."

"I love you, Eric. Come as soon as you can."

"I have to drop Johanna off at school, Hon; then I'll be there" (Aaron was already at his school).

We agreed we would talk first, before telling the kids. But Johanna's emotional antennae were on hyperalert. "Is anything wrong, Dad?" Not being very good at misdirection or mistruths, I probably hesitated just long enough for her to know that, yes, something is wrong. "What is it, Dad?"

I made a split-second decision. For better and for worse, ours is a very open house, and I was not going to start shutting her out on this. I did my best to answer her question, then called Joan to say I had let Johanna know. Joan understood. She spoke briefly with Johanna.

A few minutes later, Johanna and I were in the car, stopped in front of her school. "I don't feel like going to school. May I go to the hospital and see Mom?" Nothing would be accomplished by having Johanna sit in school. We drove to the hospital.

We entered the room, not sure of what we would hear or how Joan would be. We hugged. "Mom, I love you."

"I love you, too, Johanna."

Johanna was open with her fears. "What's going to happen? Will you be okay? Dad, what if you get sick?"

"Don't worry, honey. I promise I'll take good care of myself."

Joan's attention was focused on Johanna's need for reassurance. Joan did her best to "normalize" things. We played a few games of casino. Joan did her laps with Johanna and me. Falling into familiar parental roles, we tried to protect Johanna as best we could. But we also knew that her life was now forever changed.

I don't really remember everything that took place that day. Joan spoke with Cathy. I spoke with George, and we developed a list of questions for Dr. Brown, the first of many lists.

We met with Dr. Brown later in the day. The pathology report showed that the cancer had spread to the lymph nodes. (Seven out of thirty nodes tested positive.) But the "good news" (what constituted "good news" was already undergoing redefinition!) was that there was no evidence of spread beyond the lymph nodes. So Joan's cancer was initially staged as IIIb. In lay terms, "You're in deep sh*t, baby! But things could be worse." Joan understood, better than I, that this was not a promising diagnosis. Dr. Brown arranged for us to meet a local oncologist, Dr. Himpler, the next day.

Johanna stayed at the hospital with Joan, and I returned to Manlius to let Aaron know that his mom had cancer. Picking him up early from soccer practice, we talked, and then drove back to Crouse Hospital to be with Joan and Johanna. Aaron's concern and warmth showed in his eyes. Joan again shifted into parental reassurance mode.

Dropping the kids off at home, I went to the open house at Johanna's middle school. I remember letting the principal and Johanna's English teacher know about what was happening in our family. Not much more.

Later I returned to the hospital. Alone with me, Joan could give more expression to her fears. Why was this happening? We had both worked so hard to put a good family together. And now this! We cried, we joked (maybe this is just a bad dream?), we spoke with friends, we did some laps. I went home.

Morning came, and the kids went off to school. With my new colleagues at Syracuse University handling my classes, I could be with Joan at the hospital.

DEVELOPING A PLAN: PART I

Up until now, the cancer had had its way. Now it was time to do something about it. We began learning about treatment options, met with local oncologists, and started thinking about getting second and third opinions at major cancer centers. We also began to collect our emotions and think about the need to put supports in place for our children and for ourselves.

Stressing the need to be deliberate, George helped us develop questions for the oncologist and think about possible strategies for dealing with the disease. Our friend Madelyn Siegel Baum provided a good ear and equally good advice negotiating this new world we were entering. Another M.D. friend, a Massachusetts oncologist, counseled us to be thoughtful in our selection of an oncologist and offered to be available to us as questions came up.

Later, Dr. Himpler came into Joan's room and sat by her bed. A polite man with a dry sense of humor, we liked him. Even so, the similarity between "Himpler" and "Himmler," the name of the Gestapo chief who administered Hitler's death camps, did not escape my attention.

A plan began to take form. The standard chemotherapy—5FU and Leucovorin—seemed to be the way to go. With luck, we could knock out the cancer before it invaded any other systems. "Are there other treatments? Should we get a second opinion at Dana Farber Cancer Center in Boston, Dr. Himmler, excuse me, Dr. Himpler?" (Try as I might, "Himmler" kept breaking through my subconscious.) Dr. Himpler was open to a second opinion, but made it clear that he did not favor high-tech experimental interventions. We liked his directness. We thought it likely that we would work with him. Even so, we were still considering meeting with another oncologist, Tony Scalzo, when he returned the following week from vacation. We also decided to seek an opinion from a colon cancer specialist at a major cancer center.

George contacted several colleagues to identify the most respected colon cancer specialists in Boston and New York City. Dana Farber's Robert Mayer and Memorial Sloan-Kettering's Nancy Kemeny came out as among the very best. Having just moved from Boston, we made arrangements to meet with Dr. Mayer.

But how would we get in to see someone like Dr. Mayer? I had wrongly assumed, as I think many people do, that only the rich and famous receive care at a place like Dana Farber. I called friends who had political connections, asking if they would help us to be seen there. Turned out, all I needed to do was call Dr. Mayer's office and set up an appointment for a consultation. He was very busy, but his practice was taking appointments, although there was a wait. Thanks to Karen Kayser, yet another former colleague in Boston who was doing research at Dana Farber, and Peter Bent Brigham Hospitals, we were able to get an early appointment.

The remainder of Joan's five-day Crouse Hospital stay was filled with telephone calls from family and friends and visits from our kids. Joan kept beating a path around the hospital corridors, at first slowly, and, in a few days, closer to her normal pace though still a bit stooped. We walked, held hands, and found things to cry and laugh about. I prepared classes and Joan read novels. She walked to help speed her recovery and because being active was one of the ways she dealt with anxiety.

Joan was beginning to adjust to the harsh reality of a cancer diagnosis. She knew we were looking at an uphill battle, but she was not without hope. No question I would be with her no matter what. To do so was instinctual, but also a way for me to deal with my fear of losing her. As I would find out, going down this path with Joan and our family—while deeply sad in many ways—would be the most meaningful experience of my life, deepening our understandings of each other and of what is important in life.

We started making plans for Joan to come home. We expected that it would take a few weeks before she would be ready to do things around the house. Cathy would come from Boston to spend the first week with us. We would buy a bed frame to raise our mattress from the floor, making it easier for Joan to get in and out of bed. Joan didn't want to be fussed over, but she acceded to this $40 purchase.

Dr. Kasowitz stopped by for a short visit, one that turned out to be very memorable. He asked Joan about her plans for treatment. Responding that she had talked with Dr. Himpler and would meet Dr. Scalzo next week, she mentioned the consult we had scheduled at Dana Farber with Dr. Mayer. As Dr. Kasowitz (who we were soon calling "Mark") later said, "I almost fell off the chair." He shared with Joan that he and his wife, Ronnie, had just returned from a consult with Dr. Mayer. Unfortunately, we were all members of the same club—a club that no one wants to be part of.

Joan called to tell me how touched and appreciative she was with Mark's openness to us. In a very practical way, it helped to know that we were seeing a "doctor's doc" and to learn that Ronnie Kasowitz and Mark were working with Dr. Scalzo as their local oncologist and that Dr. Scalzo was open to working with Dr. Mayer. More importantly, Joan appreciated that Mark saw her as a person, not simply as a "cancer patient." Later, we would get to know Ronnie, another person who lived well with cancer, at chemotherapy infusions.

To completely rule out the possibility of liver metastases, a night nurse suggested to Joan that she ask for another CT scan, this time with a dye injected into her arm. The nurse told Joan of a friend who went through one form of treatment for breast cancer, only to find out several months later that the cancer was in her liver, and that she should have started with a different treatment.

When I saw Joan the following morning, she told me about the discussion, saying she hadn't slept much afterwards. Should she ask for another CT? She had had a CT one month earlier that suggested that her liver was clear. But it was done without IV contrast.

That day, Joan asked for another scan. The doctor didn't see much reason for it. Even if they found liver involvement, the treatment would probably be the same—5FU and Leucovorin. And the earlier scan suggested the liver was clear. But he ordered the scan and Joan had it the day before she was discharged.

GOING HOME

Even without any health problems, our family was undergoing lots of change. We had just moved. The kids were in new schools. I was starting a new job. And Joan would soon be looking for one, we had thought.

Nothing would ever be "normal" again, but our family life remained good.

We wanted Aaron and Johanna to be kids. We didn't want to see the cancer rob them of their teenage years. What messages to give them? We couldn't promise them that everything would be okay. But we did promise them that we wouldn't hide information from them. They wouldn't have to second-guess anything. (We kept our word.)

Like most parents, we rejoiced in seeing Aaron and Johanna enjoy themselves and do the things that kids are supposed to do—even when they were being "pains." "We don't want you to feel bad about having a good time. But don't think you have to have a good time or pretend to be having one, just to make us feel good," we advised.

The messages delivered by Joan's actions were powerful. She greatly valued maintaining the routines of our home. Coming home for the first time as a cancer patient, she hugged the kids, Cathy, and Baltimore (the family dog). Taking one look at the house (which was perfectly neat by my standards), she took the broom from the closet, and started sweeping the kitchen and family room. "Joan, come on, Hon. Take it easy," I protested. "Eric, this makes me feel good," she retorted. I shook my head, a little frustrated, but mostly proud to see this expression of her strength and love. (And, truth be told, I was probably a bit relieved that she was not asking me to clean up the house.) At times, it was frustrating to see her push herself so hard, give so much. But I also knew that this tenaciousness and commitment to maintaining our family gave meaning to her life and to ours.

I started to reestablish my teaching routines. One morning, Claire Rudolph, an older colleague, came up to me in the campus parking lot and said that Lionel, her husband, a highly regarded Syracuse internist, had a message for me. "Lionel says that this cancer can be beat; but Joan will need aggressive treatment. He said he would be pleased to meet with you." (A couple weeks later, when we met, Lionel handed me the abstracts of three studies he had pulled off the National Cancer Institute's Web site. Two of them were of experimental chemotherapies [CPT-11 (aka Ironetecan) and Oxaliplatin] that Joan later benefited from by participating in clinical trials. Both are now approved for use with metastatic colon cancer.) Claire, who had already shared with me that she was a survivor of an advanced cancer, also encouraged Joan to talk with Tony Scalzo, her oncologist and soon to be Joan's.

Deb Monahan, a colleague whose family has a history of ovarian cancer, suggested that we could learn a lot about treatment options from information available over the Internet. My friend Alejandro was always available to listen, and even held me one day when I broke down in tears in his office having learned that the prognosis for Joan's cancer was even worse than I had thought.

I started to search around the Internet for information about stage IIIb colon cancer. The numbers were not great. More than 50 percent of persons treated with the then-standard therapy—5FU (Fluorouracil) and Leucovorin—died within five years. The percentages were far worse for people with liver involvement. Joan decided right from the beginning that she did not want to hear "the numbers." They weren't good and would only scare her. Moreover, in many ways the numbers are not particularly relevant, since they are often based on studies that began ten or more years ago. As Dr. Mayer later said to me after I requested that he not discuss probabilities, "I never discuss probabilities with patients. They are not relevant. For any one individual, the probability of surviving is either 100 percent or zero."

Joan had the heavy lifting. She had to come to terms with the possibility of dying, contemplate treatment, comfort our children. We set up appointments with the guidance counselors and with a couple of teachers at the kids' schools. We stayed in close contact with our friend Faith Ball, an English teacher in the high school. Teachers were notified. Dana Pierce, our son's high school guidance counselor, and later our daughter's as well, made herself very available to both kids. And, like Faith, Dana was present through the entire illness, sharing her wisdom, smiles, and tears with all of us.

Joan started thinking about how to approach the disease. A reader, she began looking at the "Chicken Soup for the Soul" books, Bernie Siegel books, and stories of how people dealt with cancer. We both read *Healing Lessons* by Sidney Winawer, a highly regarded oncologist whose book provided insight into the paths Joan and I might take.

Very quickly, Joan rejected the idea of "fighting her cancer." She would do all that was reasonable to live, and hopefully to eliminate the cancer, but the "battling" metaphor didn't work for her. To battle cancer felt like she would be fighting herself. Instead of battling herself, the idea of learning how to better love herself took root. This was her approach. When she spoke of the possible cause of the cancer, she traced it back to Betty, her stepmother, who was such a negative force in her life. And occasionally, she would locate the cause in the stress and unhappiness she experienced as a student at the Boston College School of Nursing.

Likewise, as she read through the self-help books, she developed an aversion to the idea that people can gain control over their cancer and cure themselves. She believed strongly in the importance of dealing with the emotional aspects of the disease and with opening herself up to benefit from various treatments. She was open to western medicine, to eastern medicine, to the full range of standard and complementary therapies. But she resented what she viewed as a "blaming the victim" subtext that flowed through some of the self-help books. Yes, there probably is a psychosomatic component to many cancers. But, as she would say, some books go too far in their assumption that people can control their cancer. The truth is, she would comment, you can do everything right in dealing with this "fuck*ng" disease and still die. That shouldn't mean you failed or lost a battle. Just that you didn't live as long as you wanted.

Joan was exceptionally robust. We all anticipated that Joan's activity would be limited for several weeks as she recovered from abdominal surgery. Not so. Within a couple of days, Joan was up to her old routines—making meals, cleaning, and taking long walks with Baltimore around Green Lakes State Park and Mill Run Park.

Joan began to lay the foundation for dealing with the cancer. In the months that followed, she dealt through keeping our family and home whole, walks in the state park with Baltimore and whoever else was around, novels, quieting herself, conversations, courage, laughter, and love. These approaches would work well.

GOOD SCAR, BAD SCAN

It felt like we had begun to pick ourselves up after having been run over by a steamroller. Now we were going to find out what happens when the steamroller goes into reverse gear and gets you a second time.

Tuesday, October 13, 1998

Arriving at the now all-too-familiar Physicians Office Building on Irving Avenue in Syracuse, Cathy, Joan, and I were looking forward to seeing Dr. Brown. Dr. Brown was going to take a look at Joan's incision and possibly remove the staples. (Seems that staples are now used more than stitches.) Joan looked forward to getting them out.

Joan and I went into Dr. Brown's examination room first. Dr. Brown examined the scar line. "Looks very good. Let's get these staples out. Joanie, come to my office when you're dressed. I want to talk with you."

Now joined by Cathy, we introduced her to the new "Dennis" in our lives. Cathy would later agree that Dr. Brown resembled their brother, Dennis, both physically and in the kindness of his manner.

We were completely unprepared for what we would hear. How can you ever be prepared to hear that your life is being cut very short? With clear concern for the harsh impact of the message he was about to deliver, Dr. Brown said that the CT scan came back with some ambiguous results. "There were a couple of spots on the scan. It might be nothing, just some areas where several veins come together. But we should do a couple of tests to rule out a lesion in the liver."

With the word "liver," a shock went through my body, centering on my stomach. "This is a nightmare. Joan's going to die," I thought. Joan later told me I looked like I had been hit in the stomach with a two by four. I probably quipped, "I wish it were only that."

Again, in shock, we listened as best we could. Dr. Brown arranged for a MRI for the next day. He didn't want us to have to wait. We left, thanking him for the consideration he was showing us, and appreciative of how he had broken this news to us. We were terribly scared but still felt that things might be okay—that Joan's colon cancer might be stage IIIb, not IV. One hell of a definition of "okay"!

Wednesday, Thursday, Friday, October 14, 15, 16

The roller coaster kept heading "South." The MRI scan, read by three radiologists, was inconclusive—a split decision, with two saying the liver was probably clear, and one seeing a problem. Still hopeful that we might dodge this bullet, Dr. Brown arranged for an ultrasound. Having left one of our cars in the imaging center's parking lot, we left a note that we would pick it up in a day or two. We needed to be together.

That night, Joan and I went to the open house at Aaron's high school. In the halls, we blended in with other parents rushing about from class to class, making contact with their children's teachers and neighbors. Going through the motions of our old life was comforting, but it also highlighted how different our life had become.

The next day brought more bad news. The ultrasound results confirmed the likelihood of liver involvement. A liver biopsy was scheduled for Friday, the sixteenth.

Later that day, we had our first visit with Dr. Scalzo. A large practice, his partners have an attractively decorated office, with candy, coffee, and other foodstuffs available to patients and family members. Hematology-Oncology also provides patients access to a social worker, support groups, a nutritionist, and to nurse-practitioners who are actively involved in patient care.

A tall, dark-skinned Italian, Dr. Scalzo's Hollywood looks do not escape people who meet him. Joan talked comfortably about her views of dealing with cancer. She was prepared to do what could be done, within reason. She hoped her cancer could be treated, that she could get it in remission. But there were certain places she did not want to go. Some treatments are worse than death, she said. It was important to her to know that Dr. Scalzo would respect her boundaries, and communicate pros and cons of treatment options.

Dr. Scalzo, who soon became "Tony," was open to a Dana Farber consult, and willing to consider front-line treatments. Without knowing whether the cancer had metastasized to the liver, the treatment path wasn't clear. I asked my "what if" question. He suggested an appointment early the next week, when we would have better information. I pressed him some about what could be done if it were in the liver. I recall getting frustrated with his use of the word "palliative." There must be more that can be done.

Joan and I drove home, trying to piece together what was happening in our lives. We had worked so hard to make a good life, a good family. And now cancer seemed likely to destroy our lives. All I knew about metastases to the liver was that such a diagnosis was virtually a death sentence, one likely to be carried out very quickly. We were convinced that tomorrow's test would confirm what we already felt we knew. Joan cried. I cried. We pulled ourselves together for our kids. We were not going to hide anything from them, but made a decision not to let them know until we were sure. No point in having them go through this anxiety if it turned out that the liver was clear.

By Friday afternoon, we had the answer we already knew and never wanted to hear. There were three, possibly four lesions in the liver.

Dr. Brown explained that surgical resection of the cancer was impossible. There were too many metastases (three or four), and they were too close to a major artery. He had done liver surgery, but only when there were one or at most two lesions.

Later that night, I looked up stage IV colon cancer on the Internet. With the standard treatment—5FU and Leucovorin—Joan might have six months. Without it, maybe three. I called George from our basement, away from the ears of my family. He listened as my voice quivered, and I broke down in tears.

"Yes, this isn't good, Eric, but keep in mind that there are new treatments and the statistics are based on old studies. Let's see what Dr. Mayer says. Think about an appointment with Dr. Kemeny." George, referring again to the roller-coaster metaphor, suggested that things are rarely as bad or as good as they look on this ride. "Hang in there, Eric."

We set our sights and hopes on a meeting with Dr. Mayer, scheduled for the following Friday.

4

From Despair to Hope

$\mathscr{S}$ I cannot do justice to the emotions we experienced over the next few weeks.

Joan was preparing to die, but we were also trying to settle the family in a new community. And hoping to find some hope.

I talked with Joan about going back to Boston to be near Cathy and Mary Jo and many good friends. I called the president's office at Boston College, to see if I might come limping back to my old job. It might be possible, I was told. Joan took a "let's see" attitude, feeling that the kids were better off in their new schools, and I at mine. Besides too much was happening to contemplate a move.

Joan gave voice to not wanting to be viewed as "that poor person who came to Syracuse, got cancer, and died." She didn't want to be defined by her disease. At times she would despair, "Why don't I just die now and get it over with? It's going to happen anyway. There's nothing you or anyone else can do about this, Eric. I might as well save you a lot of trouble and be done with it."

I kept looking for reasons to hope. I spent hours searching the National Cancer Institute and other Web sites (see appendix B). I was learning more about colon cancer than I ever wanted to know. Finding studies that stretched five-year survival probabilities for Joan's type of cancer from 3 to 7 percent. Some people had to be among the 7 percent. It could be Joan. She fit the profile of a survivor.

Maybe there was an experimental drug that could push Joan's cancer into remission? After all, there were some promising lines of research. Antiangiogenesis drugs try to block the creation of new veins that feed tumors. Without a blood supply, the tumors can't grow. Better yet, they shrink and dissipate. Monoclonal antibodies seek to target tumors. The "smart bombs" of the cancer arsenal, the hope is that they will help deliver chemo directly to the cancer cells, allowing for more effective and less invasive treatment. Or some surgical procedure? But would Joan be willing to explore such possibilities if they exist? Might the treatment be worse than death? Joan was clear about wanting to maintain quality of life as long as possible. And, as noted, she felt there were things worse than death. Still, George and others reminded me that the published probability data were old. They were based on old approaches to treatment, and new drugs were coming on line all the time. If we could buy some time, then maybe one of the new approaches to treatment could help Joan and I reach old age together.

Joan and I talked with Gussie Sorensen, the social worker at Hematology-Oncology. Gussie listened as Joan described the path before her. Stretching her open hand before us, Joan said she saw three paths, the largest and most probable was that she would not live very long. A second path might include a period of remission, and the smallest path a cure. No percents here, just waves of the hand covering areas indicating the relative likelihoods. She hoped for the best, but needed to prepare for whichever path was hers. Gussie said something like, "Hope is good on this journey. You may find that hope changes as you go along." This last comment stuck with me. Thirty-two months later, as I prayed for Joan to die, I thought of Gussie's words. And, since Joan's death, these words have echoed in my mind as I try to talk with Joan.

Driving to school, I found myself crying out, "God, please don't take Joan. Give us time." I would pull over and scream out my pain and tears. I tried bargaining with God. "Take me and leave Joan." I yelled at God, "Why are you letting this happen? Please don't let her die." Somehow I managed to get through my classes.

It was hard to be away from Joan. Coming home each day, we would hold each other closely, sometimes starting to cry. Some days we would take walks at Green Lakes. Joan would walk and walk to shed some of her anxiety.

On one walk, Joan stopped and, looking at the trees and lake before us, commented, "I'm glad I haven't been an asshole. I can't imagine facing this illness thinking I had wasted my life being a jerk. I've walked softly on this earth and this feels good."

The evenings during these first few weeks were especially difficult. Dinner was often punctuated with tears. The cancer news wasn't great. "Can't we talk about something else besides cancer?" Johanna asserted with her usual directness at one meal. Aaron nodded in assent.

Joan would ask about happenings at school, soccer practices and the like, but, inevitably, the conversation came back to cancer. Trying to keep spirits alive, I might repeat some of the wisdom that friends had passed on. The kids became especially fond of one—"It's only money."

Scott and Susan Plumb, two longtime friends from Boston, visited. Having dealt with Susan's breast cancer, they knew some of what we were experiencing. Susan told the story of picking up her car after her final radiation treatment. Apologizing profusely, the hospital parking lot attendant showed her a fresh dent in the side of the car. Having faced her own morality and relieved to be done with chemo, Susan was not terribly bothered. "It's only money." Scott and Susan had adopted this mantra shortly after diagnosis. Turned out that our kids, like theirs, thought it was a pretty neat concept. "But, Dad, it's only money!"

Later that week Aaron—a newly licensed driver—had his first accident. An unlicensed driver made an illegal turn, broadsiding our 1989 Volvo wagon. Adopting Scott and Susan's mantra, Joan and I decided to cash out a portion of our pension savings for a new car with airbags. We also decided to use some of this money to make our surroundings at home pleasant (that is, purchasing some rugs, refinishing some furniture).

Reaching a decision to spend this money was difficult for Joan. Joan was not especially interested in material things, and she was more cautious about purchases than I. We had been anticipating two incomes in our home. With the cancer, that changed, and Joan was worried about our finances. But Joan accepted my argument that we would be okay. As

I put it, from a financial point of view, the worst-case scenario was that Joan would live and we would spend many years together with a slightly reduced retirement income—a wonderful outcome, as far as we were concerned. If she died, we had life insurance and it would replace the pension income. Either way, we would be fine financially. So, let's put some things in place that would make our lives more comfortable and, in the case of the new car, reduce some of the stresses in our lives.

A related piece of advice came from my cousin Jim Kramon who, along with his wife, Paula, has had enough contact with docs to last several lifetimes. Twelve years ago, Paula had a bone marrow transplant for lymphoma at Dana Farber in Boston. Lyme disease, invasive to the central nervous system, greatly restricts Jim's mobility and is a source of chronic pain. When I talked about the diagnosis with Jim, a highly regarded Baltimore lawyer with a razor-sharp wit, he referred to the experience he had making frequent visits to Boston after Paula's transplant. Paula was extremely sick, in much pain, and in an isolation room for many months. Jim stayed at a hotel in Cambridge. Every morning on his way to visit Paula, he would buy a cup of coffee and sit by the Charles River. "I realized that you can't control the big things, Eric. But you can control some of the little things, like that cup of coffee. They matter." Our "cups of coffee" came in the form of our capacity to find humor where we could, from attending the kids' athletic matches, and an occasional decision to fly rather than drive to New York City for chemotherapy.

DEVELOPING A PLAN: PART II

Strange disease! Joan might die within a couple of months, but she looked and felt fine. No one would have blamed Joan if she chose to "put her head in the sand." Fortunately, she didn't. We made plans to see Dr. Mayer in Boston and Dr. Kemeny in New York City, arranging for CT scans, surgical reports, and biopsy slides to be sent first to Dr. Mayer.

Better News at Dana Farber

Arriving at Dana Farber on October 23, we were met by Cathy and George at Dr. Mayer's office. The receptionist was welcoming and told us that there would not be much of a wait. It was just long enough, it turned out, for us to do a last-minute review of our questions. George and Cathy would be our third and fourth set of ears. We strategized that at the end of the office visit, George would see if he could get a minute with Dr. Mayer to talk "doctor to doctor."

Robert Mayer, a warm and approachable personality, came out shortly and after greeting us, asked if we would mind if he took an extra minute or two because he wanted a second radiologist to take a look at the scans. No objections from us! As he walked back to his office, I quietly asked him to give us a little hope, even if he thought there was none. "Dr. Mayer, Joan has been hit with one piece of horrible news after another. Even if you think this is a hopeless situation, it would be helpful to give us the news in a way that allows for some hope. Also, if it's okay, could you avoid talking about 'percents' with Joan. That wouldn't be helpful for her." He responded, "I never talk about percents to patients. For any individual, the 'percent' is either 100 or 0." I felt heard. "Thanks." He went to his office.

In a few minutes, he called Joan in for an exam, a very thorough one. He was very well prepared for the visit, with good recollection of Joan's medical history and scans.

He called all of us into his office. Directing his comments to Joan, he presented an option we did not anticipate. We were all taken with his warmth and his thoughtful demeanor. It might be possible to resect the liver tumors, he said. He went on to explain that liver metastases are either slow or fast growing. If Joan's were slow growing, then it would make sense to explore surgery. He advised doing nothing for the next three to six months to see whether the tumors grow. If there is not much growth, then surgery would be considered. Other treatments were possible, but this would be the most efficacious.

The consult lifted our spirit. Over lunch at the Elephant Walk in Brookline, we all agreed Dr. Mayer is "a mensch"—a competent, warm, teddy bear of a doc. Joan felt very comfortable in his and Dr. Scalzo's care. Relieved that she did not have to start chemotherapy, she decided to follow Dr. Mayer's advice. She was elated that she could go home and have the holidays. Not being disposed to leaving the kids, Joan saw no reason to seek a third opinion from Dr. Kemeny. Besides, Boston was a logical place for us to receive care if surgery was possible, and Dana Farber was an outstanding cancer center.

Returning home, we had a short respite. Dr. Mayer had given us some hope. Deciding that short-term employment or volunteer work would be a useful distraction, Joan began talking with people about opportunities. During the day, she took many walks with Baltimore around Green Lakes and Mill Run Parks. Michele visited from Baltimore. Cathy from Boston. We went to the kids' soccer games. Joan organized our lives—arranging orthodontist and pediatrician visits for Aaron and Johanna, welcoming their new friends to our house, making plans for Thanksgiving.

Friends were pleased to see a little bit of the pressure taken off all of us. Madelyn Siegel Baum was impressed that Dr. Mayer suggested not treating the disease for a while, noting that it takes courage for an oncologist to suggest not intervening. George seemed uneasy about the course of action but respectful of Joan's decision.

Second Thoughts

With the sword of Damocles clearly visible, our lives had a surreal quality. No doubt the people Joan talked with about employment were puzzled about how to respond. One colleague, meaning well, suggested she might want to volunteer for the local hospice. A poorly timed comment by Johanna's pediatrician—"Oh, what a terrible diagnosis"—sent Joan's spirits tumbling. Within a few days, Joan's anxiety rose and, as always, mine followed in tandem.

Hearing me give voice to my fear that Dr. Mayer might just be doing what I had requested—giving us a little hope—our friend the Massachusetts oncologist suggested keeping the Dr. Kemeny option open. "She's a very different personality from Dr. Mayer, but equally committed and respected. Her approach may be more aggressive. You just might want to see what she says." Good advice. I got off the phone and called George, asking him to set up the appointment with Dr. Kemeny at Sloan.

In retrospect, the period between our consult with Dr. Mayer and our first meeting with Dr. Kemeny seemed like forever. But it was only ten days.

The appointment was set for November 2. One of my social work students, Deb Livingston, was willing to stay at our home with the kids while we were away. We met with Deb. The chemistry was good. Deb didn't want to be paid, but we insisted otherwise.

We drove to New York City, cherishing the wonderful friend we had in each other. Joan's hands held my free hand tightly for much of the trip. I told her how much I love her. We drove.

George's mother, Peggy Igel, opened her home to us. I have known and liked Peggy ("Mrs. Igel") forever—that is, since George and I became friends in 1959. Staying in her home was comforting. No need for formalities with Peggy. We lapped up the surrogate mothering on this and many subsequent stays.

Arriving around dinnertime, we went to George and Ronnie Igel's home for dinner (George and his mother lived in the same building). After dinner, George, Joan, and I prepared questions for the meeting with Dr. Kemeny. Dr. Kemeny, George reminded us, had a very different style from Dr. Mayer. Not warm and fuzzy, but equally well-regarded and a very strong advocate for her patients. We became very close to her over the next thirty months.

Sloan-Kettering: A Different Perspective

Dr. Kemeny is internationally known for her work with colon cancer that has metastasized to the liver. Because the liver rids the blood of poisons and other waste products, it is a difficult organ to treat with systemic chemotherapy. Standard doses of chemotherapy are often too low to have much of an effect on the liver. More concentrated doses might be more effective in treating the liver but are also likely to kill far too many healthy cells in other organs. Dr. Kemeny has pioneered a way of delivering a more concentrated level of chemo directly to the liver, thereby avoiding high doses to the other organs since the liver first detoxifies the chemo before it flows to other organs. The gall bladder is removed and a heat-activated refillable pump—about the size of a hockey puck—is implanted. The chemotherapy agent is injected into a chamber of the pump and released slowly. The pump is refilled monthly, sometimes with chemotherapy and other times with glycerin, designed to keep the pump from getting clogged.

I had read abstracts showing modest increases (a few months) in length of survival for persons with unresectable liver metastases when the pump was used. A few months didn't seem like much. But the five-year survival rates (23 percent) for patients selected to participate in Dr. Kemeny's clinical studies that combined liver surgery, implantation of the pump, and systemic chemotherapy were dramatic.

Arriving at Sloan the next morning, Joan and I made our way to Dr. Kemeny's office area. The day was in full swing. About forty people—patients and family members—crowded into a waiting room, each with their own story and fears. Mentioning that Dr. Kemeny was running behind schedule, the receptionist asked Joan to fill out some paperwork. We waited. George joined us. We waited some more. Joan talked about how much she feared and disliked the idea of having a pump implanted. We played some cards. We waited. Joan's name was called.

We were ushered into a small examination room. A young doctor breezed in. No bedside manner, just a "Hello, I'm Dr. Kemeny's fellow, and I'd like to ask you a few questions." He began the interview, only stopping to assert what a great place Sloan is and how we had come to the right place. (I felt like telling him to screw off but kept my thoughts to myself.)

Dr. K's fellow left the room, and Joan and George and I laughed about how this experience was shaping up to be a lot different from the one we had at Dana Farber. "I can tell already I think I'll want to work with Dr. Mayer."

Dr. Kemeny entered the room a few minutes later. After short introductions, she said something like, "Alright, tell me why you're here and what you have been told." Joan repeated the story, saying she had been advised that the liver tumors might be resectable, but that she should wait three to six months to see whether they were slow or fast growing. Reflexively, Dr. K. shot back, "Who said that?" Joan indicated that she had consulted with Dr. Mayer. "I know Bob. We've done some research together. He's a very good doctor, but I couldn't disagree with him more on this. If these mets can be resected, then they should be taken out. It doesn't matter if they are slow or fast growing. You're a young person, so they probably are growing more quickly. But, either way, if we can get them out, it's to your advantage. I understand where Bob is coming from, but I disagree with his approach. It would make more sense to me if he starting chemotherapy while you were waiting. But even if he had suggested that, I would disagree with this approach." Picking up Joan's CT scans, she said, "Let me take a look at these again. I'll be right back." Exit Dr. K.

Initially, Dr. Kemeny's style rubbed me the wrong way. My first impression was that, though perhaps brilliant, she was not the right person for us. How wrong I was! In time, Joan and I would develop a very trusting and friendly relationship with Dr. Kemeny. But, as I told Dr. Kemeny several years later, right then I had to bite my tongue. I am very glad that I did.

Joan and I didn't know what to make of this first encounter. One of us might have quipped, "Well, she's not warm and fuzzy!"

Dr. Kemeny returned, saying that she thought the liver might be resectable. She wanted to show the scans to Dr. Yuman Fong as soon as he was out of surgery. Could we wait and possibly meet with him today or tomorrow? We were dazed. We really did not understand what all this meant. Joan mentioned she did not want to initiate a treatment that would undermine her quality of life. Dr. Kemeny responded, "It's usually the tumors, not the treatments, that undermine quality"—words whose wisdom I came to appreciate.

As we had previously agreed, George asked to speak privately with Dr. Kemeny. Returning to the examination room, George said, "This may be very good news." The thought crossed my mind that George was just trying to keep our spirits up. It was hard to see how the possibility of having most of your liver taken out could be good news. Or, how having two of the world's leading oncologists giving you diametrically opposed opinions could qualify as "good news." But, as we would learn, it was good news.

Late in the day, we met Dr. Fong, a short man in his mid-thirties. A good listener and patient communicator, he did not fit the stereotype of a surgeon. Yes, he thought the liver might be resectable, but would want to have a dynamic CT scan done at Sloan before making a decision to do surgery. One of the mets was very close to the vena cava, so he would need to see whether there was sufficient room. Joan would need to come back to Sloan next week. She would be sedated. A small incision would be made in the groin, and a catheter inserted through an artery directly into the liver, allowing for a dye to be injected in a manner that provided a better view of the positioning of the metastases.

The following day, Joan took the next step, telling Dr. Kemeny that she had decided to have the dynamic CT scan. It was scheduled for November 9.

Driving to Syracuse, the conversation turned to the contradictory recommendations we had received. Dr. Brown and Dr. Scalzo had said that the metastases were not resectable. Dr. Mayer, that they might be, but that Joan should wait. Dr. Kemeny and Dr. Fong that they might be and that, if so, Joan should not wait. We were not surprised that highly specialized doctors might recommend interventions that local docs considered infeasible. But we were not prepared for the Mayer/Kemeny split. We felt more comfortable with Dr. Mayer's style, but the idea of waiting to see whether the tumors would grow and kill Joan was not appealing. Of course, the alternative—a five- to seven-hour surgery in which two-thirds of your liver would be taken out—wasn't all that comforting either. Anyway, no decisions needed to be made right away.

We discussed our children, and how they were handling everything. For Joan, who had lost her own mother when young, the thought of leaving Aaron and Johanna was unbearable. We listened to the music from *Les Misérables,* which seemed to give expression to the depths of the feelings we were experiencing. Joan cried as Fantine, preparing to die, sings to her little daughter Cosette. I cried as Valjean promises Fantine that he will love, raise, and protect Cosette. We held hands for much of the drive.

The week passed. We went to Aaron and Johanna's soccer games. Cathy drove up for the weekend and stayed, while we drove, once again, to New York City. It was late fall. The colors were muted. Some trees were now bare. We were listening to music. A half hour out of Syracuse, a James Taylor song, "You've Got a Friend," played, precipitating a long cry. "I'm going to leave so much. We've worked so hard, Eric. It just doesn't seem right that this is happening. Why are we bothering to do this? I'm just going to die anyway. Why don't I just go home and take whatever time is left with the kids?" We held hands, talked about how much we loved each other and our kids—how proud we were of the family we had put together. She cried much of the way to New York City, mourning the life she expected to lose, and fearing the interventions that might keep her alive.

We arrived early for day surgery. After signing forms indicating that she understood that all sorts of horrible things might happen in this otherwise fairly benign procedure, Joan put on hospital garb and got on the hospital gurney. We were very nervous. We waited, playing casino and listening to a mother and daughter squabble behind the curtain that separated them from us. It helped pass the time.

A nurse talked with Joan about the procedure and hooked her up to an IV. Soon a tall, friendly hospital attendant, wearing a gold chain around his neck, was wheeling Joan down Sloan's long halls to the day surgery holding area. Joan was placed next to her worst fear, a heavily sedated older Caucasian woman, thin as a rail and yellowed from jaundice. She was moaning. Her husband seemed confused, not knowing what to do.

Joan would later comment, "I don't want to be one of those 'yellow people.'" But right then, she voiced annoyance that this woman shouldn't be left in pain. Her husband shouldn't have to be wandering around trying to get someone's attention. Later, at Joan's urging, I spoke with the floor administrator, who seemed genuinely concerned about what had transpired.

Dr. Karen Brown came by, and introduced herself as the radiologist who would be doing the procedure. Then George, a surgical aid, came in, announcing with a disarming smile that he would be with Joan throughout the procedure. Asking if he could draw the curtains, he announced that his first task was to shave the area on Joan where the catheter would be inserted. The thought crossed my mind that I really didn't like the prospect of some guy I don't know shaving Joan's pubic hair. I laughed at myself. Would it be better if it were some guy I knew?

Joan, visibly nervous, was wheeled into the hallway, outside the treatment room. A surgical nurse engaged her in conversation. I watched as the nurse leaned over and kissed Joan's forehead, a spontaneous act of kindness that was greatly appreciated.

I waited. Dr. Brown came out. Everything went well. I asked what she found. The possibility of resecting the liver seemed promising, she replied, but we would need to talk with Dr. Fong and Dr. Kemeny.

Later that day, Dr. Fong reviewed the findings and treatment options. Yes, if the liver could be resected, it was possible that Joan could live cancer free. His and Dr. Kemeny's research was showing substantial benefits for patients who participated in their trials (resection, pump, and systemic chemo). Even without the pump, liver surgery might result in a cure (defined as five years free of cancer.) There was one complicating factor. There was an uncharacteristic split in Joan's hepatic artery that limited the potential efficacy of the pump. Alternatively, he proposed trying to connect the pump to the mesenteric artery, but he would not know whether this could be done until he was engaged in the surgery.

Our questions poured forth. "What are the risks of dying during the surgery?" I asked.

"In my hands, about 1 percent. The liver doesn't regenerate for another 2 to 3 percent of the patients." "What do you mean regenerate?" I asked. The liver is a remarkable organ, we learned. It generally grows back in about a month. But "if you are among the unfortunate few for whom it doesn't, then you do not live." He gave us an article on which he was lead author, a state-of-the-art review of liver surgery, prognostic factors, and related treatments for patients with metastatic colon cancer (see Abstract in appendix B).

That night we prepared a list of questions for Dr. Kemeny. What chemotherapy would she use? Likely side effects? Would she be willing to coordinate care with Dr. Scalzo so that we did not have to drive to Sloan each week? How long would Joan be at Sloan? Recovery time from surgery? Would Joan's activities be permanently restricted? If Joan wanted to have the surgery, but not the pump, could this be arranged? What does it mean to participate in a trial?

Dr. Kemeny's Clinical Trial

We returned with George to Dr. Kemeny's office the next morning. As before, the waiting room was crowded. Joan was very nervous. Having most of her liver taken out did not trouble her as much as having a pump implanted.

While there, I met Barry Kearns, a thirty-five-year-old school bus driver, whose first symptoms of stage IV colon cancer appeared during his honeymoon. He was there for his six-month follow-up with Dr. K. His liver had been resected, a pump implanted, and he had endured the rigors of the six-month cycle of chemotherapy. Couldn't play in his softball league, but he was back to work part-time, enjoying being with the kids again. He was meeting with Dr. Kemeny to get the results of his most recent CT scan. Grateful to be alive, he gave expression to a sense that God was giving him time to do some good. If so, then placing Barry in our path was part of God's plan.

I asked Barry about Dr. Kemeny. "She's okay. She knows her stuff. Hard to get information out of her, though." I mentioned that Joan was very nervous about the possibility of having a pump implanted. Would he be willing to talk with her about his experience? They talked for fifteen minutes, during which Barry made a point to show her the outline of the pump under his shirt. "No big deal. Hardly know it's there."

Joan's name was called. Dr. Kemeny was joined by her research associate, Deirdre Sullivan, a young woman who had just completed college and was thinking about a research career. Together with George, we listened as Dr. Kemeny described the clinical trial that Joan would later agree to participate in.

This new trial was very similar to the Kemeny studies we had read about. The main differences involved the use of a new, smaller pump and the substitution of CPT-11 (Ironetecan) for 5FU, the standard colon cancer chemotherapy. (CPT-11 has since received FDA approval for treatment of metastatic colon cancer.) As in her other studies, the pump would be filled alternately with FUDR (Floxuridine), a chemotherapy that is closely related to 5FU, and heparin, an anti-coagulant designed to protect the pump when it was not delivering chemotherapy. The plan was for Joan to undergo six one-month cycles of chemotherapy—three weeks of CPT-11 delivered intravenously once a week, followed by one week off, and two weeks of FUDR, followed by two weeks of heparin.

In advance of meeting with Dr. Kemeny, Joan and I had learned that there were three types of clinical trials. Phase I studies were designed to simply test whether a new drug or procedure was safe. In terms of drugs, the goal of these studies was to determine the maximum safe dosage. These studies often bring people in at different dose levels, or alternatively, start with low dosages for individuals, raising dosages in small increments. Phase II studies are designed to determine whether the intervention or new drug has any positive effect at all. Phase I determines safe dosages and phase II, whether these safe dosages have any efficacy. Phase III studies test a new drug or intervention against the standard protocol. The question under investigation concerns whether the new procedure is more efficacious than the standard protocol.

Dr. Kemeny was proposing that Joan participate in a phase I/II study. Even though the new Metronics pump was in use in Canada and other similar pumps were used in the United States, this part of Dr. Kemeny's study was considered phase I. Similarly, even though CPT-11 was already in wide use in Europe, its use was considered part of a phase II study.

There were some advantages of participating in a phase I/II study.

There was already some good evidence about the efficacy of these interventions, and since this study did not require random assignment, we could be sure that Joan, if she so chose, would get front-line interventions.

Dr. Kemeny discussed the study further and then left us with Deirdre to describe the informed consent. We said we would review the materials and get back to them within a couple of days.

We left. On the way out, we saw Barry. He greeted us with a big smile. His liver was clear. No need for chemo.

Driving once again to Syracuse, Joan mentioned that she had absorbed so much bad news that she almost couldn't bear to think there was a possibility that she might live.

Joan had to make a decision—risk surgery or risk waiting. She would choose wisely. And by doing so we would learn that living with hope trumped the alternative. But this doesn't mean it was easy.

LIVING THE PLAN

Immersion in cancer health care was intense. Our fears, hopes, and emotions rose and fell with each treatment. Quiet pleasures of home and friendships and being involved in our children's lives made this painful road possible to travel.

Intensity of Interventions

The next thirty months were filled with all sorts of medical interventions. Two major and two minor surgeries: a four-hour liver resection at Sloan on December 2, 1998; a twelve-hour surgery and heated chemotherapy wash at Memorial Hospital in Worcester, Massachusetts, on July 17, 2000, to clean out abdominal metastases; a one-hour surgery using a radio frequency ablation technique at Sloan on September 12, 2000, to burn out a couple of small liver metastases; and a short surgery at Syracuse's Crouse Hospital on April 13, 2001, to insert a tube in Joan's stomach, which had been blocked by the cancer. There were short hospital stays and trips to emergency rooms and a March 2000 consultation in Winston-Salem, North Carolina. CT scans, PET scans, ultrasounds, chest X-rays, and MRIs—enough to enrich radiologists everywhere.

These months were also filled with chemotherapies: CPT-11 / FUDR from January to July 1999, Dexamethasone (Dex) from January to February 1999, Oxaliplatin and CPT-11 from October 1999 to March 2000, Xeloda from March to June 2000 and again from August to October 2001, CPT-11 and 5FU from October 2001 to April 2001. Regular blood draws, shots to raise hemoglobin and white blood cell levels, IV fluids to prevent dehydration, IV nutrients, Kytril for chemotherapy-induced nausea, Ativan for anxiety and nausea, tegafur to protect the liver, Immodium and tincture of opium for chemotherapy-induced diarrhea, and much more . . .

I spent hundreds of hours in front of the computer seeking information about new drugs and other promising interventions. We spent hundreds of hours traveling back and forth to appointments in Syracuse, New York City, Worcester, and Winston-Salem. And we both made countless calls to our health insurance company and health care providers—averaging three to six hours in most weeks.

Riding the Roller Coaster

The roller-coaster metaphor held.

After liver surgery at Sloan in November 1998, I e-mailed friends, greatly relieved that the surgery went well. With pride and some relief, a few days later I told them that Joan was up to her old tricks of taking regular walks and doing too much for everyone else.

One of the most difficult periods came in late January and early February when Joan first began chemotherapy. The CPT-11 infusions were hard on her body, but it was the Dexamethasone—added to her pump to help protect the liver and offset some of the nausea and energy drain of chemotherapy—that almost drove her crazy. Literally. Joan was far too full of energy and jittery the day or so after she would get the drug, an amphetamine. She would then crash and get quite depressed, to the point of despair. "It's not worth it, Eric. I'm going to die anyway," she said as we walked our dog in the schoolyard across from our home. "I hate this. Absolutely hate this." Thankfully, Joan went off the Dexamethasone within a couple of weeks and her spirits improved immediately.

At about this time Joan—often accompanied by me—began meeting regularly with Ann Cross, a social worker. Her office provided a calm space to reflect upon fears, sorrows, and hopes. Ann supported Joan as she explored new ways of living and valuing her life's journey and both of us as parents and best friends under great stress. Later, she would support me as I began piecing together life after Joan's death.

While Joan was participating in Dr. Kemeny's trial, from January through May 1999 we drove back and forth to New York frequently. Once the Dex was jettisoned, this became a relatively hopeful period, though certainly very challenging, especially for Joan whose body was under assault by the chemotherapy. Come June, a CT scan showed no evidence of cancer. Joan seemed as if she might be in remission. Maybe Joan would be among the 23 percent who survive at least five years, we hoped. Regardless, she felt good enough to take on two small consulting projects, one a study of access to prenatal care in Syracuse for non-English-speaking women and the other a smoking-cessation study. We enjoyed a month in our Adirondack home. But even this period of remission was not without worry because a July CT scan raised questions about a cyst on Joan's ovary.

By October 6, 1999, I was e-mailing our friends that Joan's CT scan of two weeks ago showed some "suspicious findings" (that's a euphemism in the world of colon cancer for "you're probably in some deep #&*#$"). A biopsy a week later confirmed what we suspected, that there were some tumors in the abdominal area—very small but there nonetheless. Joan started another experimental treatment—a combination of Oxaliplatin and CPT-11. "Joan looks and feels great," I reported. "It's a crazy disease and bizarre to be told your life is at risk when you feel so good! She is out doing her three-mile walk around Green Lakes, with her sister Catherine, who came for a visit."

The tumors shrank and Joan became a candidate for a special "de-bulking" surgery eventually scheduled for July 16, 2000, in Worcester, Massachusetts. By the time of her surgery, Joan's stomach was greatly distended, giving her the appearance of being five to six months pregnant. She was also in considerable pain from the tumors pressing

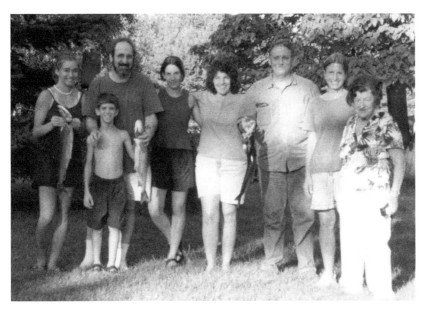

Living well: family gathering in the Adirondacks, summer 1999. From left: Maria Wolman, Matthew Kingson, Eric Kingson, Johanna Kingson, Sophie Glasgow Kingson, Steve Kingson, Joan Kingson, and Elvie Lorig.

against other organs and nerves, making it difficult for her to maintain her walking.

Still she was pleased that we were moving toward surgery because it offered relief and even hope for many more years. Joan's worst fear was that the surgeon, Dr. Swanson, would open her up and determine that there was too much spread to do anything. And she voiced fears of what shape this aggressive surgery might leave her in and of the pain she might have to endure before dying. My worst fears included Joan's but also extended to concern that she might die on the table or shortly after the surgery. I didn't want to lose her. As planned, Dr. Swanson excised as many of the tumors as possible and then soaked the abdomen for two hours with a special heated chemotherapy wash designed to treat any residue of the cancer. I prayed and worried during the surgery and after, but felt comfortable in our decision, whatever the outcome. She came through the surgery very well.

Twelve days later, I was pleased to tell friends that she had a great first night out of the hospital. "It was good to trade off tubes, 10:00 P.M. meds, 5:30 A.M. visits from the docs for long showers, dinner with friends outside on the hotel's patio, and a real bed. . . . It will take some time for Joan to recover her strength and pick up some weight, but there is every reason to think this will come with time (a couple of months)."

It did. Joan recovered quickly enough that we were able to spend a week at our summer home—an occurrence that seemed only a remote possibility two months earlier. If all went well, Joan would go back to Worcester in October to have follow-up surgery to reverse her ileostomy and clean out any cancer that remained. But the roller coaster took a sharp drop. On October 21, I wrote to friends:

T. S. Eliot was wrong. October, not April, is the cruelest month. Or at least it seems so to us. As some of you know, Joan was scheduled to have major surgery on October 17 in Worcester. Unfortunately, the PET and CT scans showed that surgery was ill-advised because there had been too much growth in the tumor since July. We were given this news in an exceptionally sensitive way, but it was hard to digest nonetheless. The bottom line—because the illness was not sufficiently contained by last summer's surgery/intrasurgical chemo wash, surgery does not make the kind of sense that systemic chemotherapy does right now.

The following Wednesday, we met with Dr. Kemeny, Joan's oncologist in NYC. She and Dr. Scalzo (Joan's oncologist in Syracuse) started Joan on a chemotherapy on Friday in Syracuse. Not a lot of fun, but it is a promising chemo because Joan has previously responded to some of the drugs that are being used. Dr. Kemeny also has two other chemo options as fallbacks, and there are some more experimental protocols that may be available in the spring.

Well, that's life in the oncological "fast lanes."

Options notwithstanding, this news was devastating. We still hoped that the chemotherapy might control the cancer, giving us additional time until another treatment became available. However, we also knew—Joan more than me—that it was improbable that even with Joan's strong will to live, that she would be able to hold back the cancer.

Joan's health continued to decline. I e-mailed friends on April 13:

I recall beginning one of my notes by saying that T. S. Eliot was wrong about April being the cruelest month. Well, it's April, and I am sorry to say that perhaps he was correct.

There have been good times during the past few months, but, overall, this has been a difficult period. In December we learned that the chemo Joan was on was not doing as much as we had hoped. In mid-January, Joan switched to another chemo. [She] is scheduled to start a new—and fairly promising experimental chemo (C-225)—next week.

About seven weeks ago, she became seriously dehydrated and lost a lot of weight due to the cumulative effects of the chemo. Since then, . . . there have been improvements, but each step forward seems to be accompanied by three-fourths of a step in the other direction and so the progress is very slow and she is fairly drained. . . . Right now she is in the hospital to deal with this weight loss and a related condition that has caused it. The goal is to get her feeling more comfortable and a bit stronger for the chemo.

So, that's it for now, except to say that in spite of how difficult these past few years have been, we are very grateful for the time and the chance to see our children do so well and to care so much for each other and feel the warmth and genuine concern of friends, family, and the many involved in Joan's care.

This was followed by a May 13, 2001, note to friends that Joan had died.

Worth Living

Joan's perseverance and good medicine added months, possibly a couple of years, to her life. She made good use of this extra time. While life was entirely changed, it continued on at our home relatively unchanged. The cancer forced us to go places that couples do not want to go, certainly not in middle age. It deepened our ties to one another and to our marriage even as it rendered physical bonds more fragile. Joan became more aware, I think, of her self-worth. We found much to celebrate in our daily life, especially Aaron's and Johanna's ability to handle themselves so well in the midst of this illness. Our children were a source of strength, pride, and great satisfaction. I wrote to friends during this time:

> Obviously, both kids are carrying a lot on their shoulders. Even so, they are managing to maintain a teenage life and stay close to us. They are warm but in different ways. Johanna is always checking in to see how Joan and I are feeling. Aaron expresses his concern in different ways, over ping pong and sometimes over quiet time spent with Joan. (No such thing as quiet time spent with Johanna! But there is much good time.)

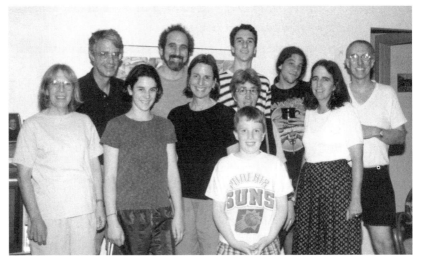

Living well: family gathering, 1999. Top row from left: Dennis Fernbach, Eric Kingson, Aaron Kingson, Peter Fernbach, Scott Veling. Middle row: JoEllen Fernbach, Johanna Kingson, Joan Kingson, Catherine Fernbach, Mary Jo Veling. Front: Michael Veling. Photograph courtesy of Alejandro Garcia.

Thankfully, our cancer years were also filled with life and lessons about the importance of living with humor, kindness, courage, and hope. Joan kept walking, our home remained warm and open to friends and family, and Aaron and Johanna seemed to thrive in their new community. There was sadness and fear, but the humor, kindness, and courage kept us from despair.

5

Kindness, Courage, and Humor in Cancer's Way

෴ Some funny, kind, and courageous things happened on the way to the oncologist. The kindness and courage of family, friends, neighbors, patients, nurses, doctors, parking lot attendants, secretaries, and even insurers helped us navigate rough patches. Like flowers growing through cracks in a sidewalk, the humor that cropped up in unexpected places enriched us.

KINDNESS

A Gift from the Parking Lot Attendant

We parked both of our cars in the lot of Syracuse's imaging center on October 14, 1998, the day Joan had her MRI to diagnose whether the cancer had spread to the liver. After the scan, we brought the films and radiologist's reports to Dr. Brown's office. He scheduled an ultrasound for the next day. While still hoping that we would get good results, we were quite sure that we wouldn't. Wanting to be together, we left a note on one of our cars in the parking lot—"Had to leave car overnight because of medical problem. Have placed $3.00 in envelope to cover costs for night & tomorrow morning. Thank you. Eric Kingson 682-xxxx."

When we picked the car up—two days, one ultrasound, and one liver biopsy later—we found a note under the windshield wiper that made us smile—a note I still carry in the glove compartment. "Good

Luck. My thoughts and prayers are with you. Bob All-Right Parking."
We wrote a short note to Bob, a middle-aged man with long hair who
looked like he had not had everything easy in life. We thanked him for
his kindness and said that his words were especially appreciated by us.

A month or so later, I stopped by to say "thank you" in person.
Bob—whose full name I later learned is Bob Corp—said he could tell we
were getting some difficult news. Showing him the note, I said that receiving it at that time meant a lot to us, and that we now carry it in the
glove compartment of our car. He laughed, pointing to a piece of paper
tacked onto the inside of the 3' by 4' enclosure that served as his office.
"See this? It's your note."

A year or so later, I stopped by to say hello again. During the conversation, he said, "You know why I have this long hair? When it gets
long enough, I have it cut off for the kids in the cancer center at University Hospital."

Liver Surgery at Sloan

December 2, 1998, was a long day, starting with Joan going into
Sloan's surgery area early in the morning and ending with George and
me seeing her at 11:30 P.M. in the postoperative care center. While waiting for the surgery, Joan and I talked, held hands. I was asked to leave
around 11:00 A.M. as they moved her into the surgical holding area. I
was comfortable being by myself. With other friends and family of patients undergoing surgery, I waited in the hospital's high-anxiety area,
reading some and making calls on my cell phone. I made a number of
visits to the hospital's chapel. Throughout the day, I would try talking
with God, deceased relatives, pets, angels—any spirit that might listen.
(I had become, and remain very open, to mysteries surrounding life. I
find strength and peace in my belief that we are more than the flesh—
though, try as I do, I cannot say that I have insights about which I am
certain.)

Dr. Fong planned to remove two-thirds of Joan's liver and implant a
pump to deliver chemo directly to the remaining liver. The pump was a
long shot because of Joan's unusual venous structure. I was surprised

by how calm—relatively speaking—I felt during much of the day. I was nervous, at first, about whether Dr. Fong would decide to go forward with the surgery. Besides losing Joan "on the table," my worst fear was that Dr. Fong would determine that the cancer was too far along for surgery to proceed. I found peace in the thoughts that we were in the hands of God, no matter what may come, and that we had made the right decision—even if Joan died during this surgery.

Learning that the surgery was definitely going forward, I relaxed a bit and went out to eat, sneaking into the cafeteria across the street at the Rockefeller Institute. I returned. More waiting. I talked with some other people who had been in the waiting area most of the day. I waited. George joined me around 5:00 or so. By 6:30 we learned that Dr. Fong was through the main part of the surgery and that it had gone well. Relief and more telephone calls followed. A little later we met with Dr. Fong in his crowded office. He was sorry the surgery got started later than planned but his morning surgery went seven hours. This tired doctor took pleasure in telling us that he was able to remove the portions of the liver that contained the metastases and maintain acceptable margins of good tissue. And he had managed to implant the pump by jerry-rigging it to a smaller vein. The company, Metronics, had shipped a special smaller shunt to him that he whittled down while in surgery to make the necessary connections possible. Lots of questions, but the bottom line: Joan was alive, and there was a good chance that the pump would work. He would go back to supervise the completion of the surgery, and then Joan would be brought to the postoperative care unit. We could see her for a few minutes in an hour or two.

Relieved and very appreciative, I thanked him. I think George commented, "Another mensch." If he didn't, he was thinking it. I certainly was.

A couple hours later, we were sitting outside the post-op unit. Picking up the wall phone, I asked if we could see my wife. "Yes, but only for a minute or two." George had warned me that Joan's appearance might be frightening. I was glad he did, because she looked ashen, almost as lifeless as my mother looked when I identified her body at the New York City coroner's office after she had died in surgery.

I was told that I could hold her hand. "I love you, Hon. You've done well." Joan smiled and mumbled a few inaudible words. I kissed her on the forehead and told her I would see her the next day.

We left. George turned to me and said, "She looks good, Eric." I responded, "If that's 'good,' I hate to think what 'bad' is." We laughed. I was comforted by George's comment and very pleased he had seen Joan with me. Otherwise, I would have been terrified. Relieved and a bit giddy, we may have repeated a little cheer we had worked up—"Scalzo, Scalzo he's our doc, if he can't do it Kemeny can. Kemeny, Kemeny, she's our doc, if she can't do it Fong can. Fong, Fong, he's our doc, if he can't do it . . ."

I went back to George's home and managed to get some reasonable sleep. Awakening once at about 5:00 A.M., I called Joan's nurse and learned that Joan was doing well. "Would you like to speak with her? We were just talking a bit. She's groggy, but I think she'd like it." Joan asked about the surgery and was relived to hear that Fong was pleased with the outcome. She told me that she vaguely recalled a dream—she didn't think it was real—that Dr. Fong or someone who looked like him visited her, wearing a baseball cap and jacket. But we learned the next day it was Fong! He had checked on Joan at 3:30 A.M. And, yes, he was a Mets fan and proud to wear their emblems. We were amazed. After two major surgeries—seven- and four-hour surgeries—he had the energy and commitment to look in on his patients in the middle of the night!

During admissions we had asked for a private room so that I could stay with Joan—strengthening our case by mentioning that we were from Syracuse and this would allow us to avoid an expensive hotel bill. A bit of a lie, since I had a place to stay either at George's or his mother's apartment. No promises, but they would try.

Later that day Joan was brought to her room—a private one—on the seventeenth floor of Sloan. Not surprisingly, she slept a lot, though as I recall, they did get her up for a short walk. She made steady and quick progress. A few days, and, by now, a couple of miles of corridor walking into her stay, Dr. Fong was able to assure us that her liver was growing back, and that the pump was working, even better than expected. The outlook? Well, we'll see. Some of the prognostic indicators are good (that is, her general health, the margins we were able to get around the tumors), some not so good (that is, the simultaneous diagnosis of her metastases and colon cancer). Discharging us one week after the surgery, he advised that we stay close to Sloan for a week. "Go see some theater or some movies. Don't worry if you feel you have to leave in the middle of a show. Just consider it a victory that you sat through some of it. Enjoy yourself. This is why I do these surgeries."

Having previously brought our bags and various accouterments to Peggy Igel's apartment, we were carrying very little when we got into the cab. On the way to Peggy's, Joan asked the cab driver to let us out on the East Side. We walked the rest of the way—about two miles—to Peggy's apartment.

Managing Managed Care

Dr. Scalzo, Joan's oncologist in Syracuse, was reading a draft of the letter from Dr. Kemeny seeking approval from our insurer to extend reimbursement for Joan's treatment at Sloan. "Nancy writes one hell of a good letter," Tony commented. We laughed. Yes, she probably does write a fine letter, we said, but we drafted much of what she put down in her letter (see the November 4, 1999, memo in appendix B).

We spent hundreds of hours negotiating the bill-paying aspects of the health care system. Realizing it was easier to avoid reimbursement problems than to fix them, we worked closely with Dr. Scalzo, Dr. Kemeny, Dr. Swanson, secretaries, nurses, and many others to craft requests in language that insurers would find acceptable (see appendix B). One trick was to avoid the word "experimental." Another required pointing out how the care Joan received outside the region of our health plan was both necessary and not available in central New York.

Of course, this strategy would not have worked if the doctors and systems we were dealing with were not open to partnering with us. Janice Livingston, the secretary in Dr. Scalzo's office, often championed our requests for CT scans and other necessary appointments. Her and other people's openness to taking our scheduling needs into consideration made difficult times a little easier. Likewise, the care and consideration of nurses like Hematology-Oncology's Sue Byrns, Crouse Hospital's Terry Principato, and Sloan-Kettering's Karen Ragusa made the "intolerable" more tolerable.

And while dealing with authorizations, billings, and bureaucratic problems was exceptionally annoying at times, for the most part the insurance company—Blue Cross Blue Shield of Central New York—and its employees and medical billing department personnel were helpful. Here, as elsewhere, persistence paid off. It was necessary to "dot your Is and cross your Ts." And, even so, we had to spend several hours each week trying to avoid or fix problems.

One particularly frightening problem arose the Friday before Joan was scheduled for Monday morning abdominal surgery (July 17, 2000) at the University of Massachusetts's Memorial Hospital. As previously mentioned, Joan's abdominal tumors had been shrunk sufficiently to allow for a possibly curative and highly unusual ten- to twelve-hour surgery performed by only ten or so surgeons in the nation. Originally scheduled and approved for Dallas, Texas, with another surgeon, we rescheduled to Worcester, Massachusetts, with Dr. Swanson. Joan had prepared herself emotionally, but she was not in good physical shape. Her tumor markers suggested that the cancer was growing again, and she had a massive amount of fluid (ascites) in her abdomen, making her appear pregnant. It was clear that some intervention was needed quickly.

Friday night at 5:00, I received a tearful telephone call from Joan. She had just learned from Dr. Swanson that our insurance company had called him at 4:45 to say that they would not fund part of the surgery because they considered it experimental. He felt caught between a rock and a hard place. He had scheduled the OR for ten hours and had arranged for ten people to be involved with various aspects of the surgery. He believed Joan needed the surgery now. He was willing to go ahead and "eat some of the cost." But he didn't think it was fair of the insurance company to put him or us in this financial predicament. It was enough to be contemplating this surgery. He would do whatever Joan wanted to do. He asked her to call me and get back to him with a decision.

Joan was conflicted, knowing she needed the surgery, and not wanting to put our family finances at risk. The decision was a no-brainer as far as I was concerned. From the beginning of the illness, we had gone for the best possible care. Until now, the insurer hadn't balked. We would ask Dr. Swanson to go forward with the surgery and fight the insurance war later. Calmer, but still upset, she hung up the phone and called Dr. Swanson.

I called Blue Cross Blue Shield of Central New York. "Hello and thank you for calling Blue Cross Blue Shield. To assure that you receive the highest quality of service, your call may be monitored. . . . Our office is closed, please listen carefully for all options. . . . For urgent requests requiring authorization within twenty-four hours, please. . . ." I followed the instructions and received some nameless person who staffed the after-hours answering service. But, as I was soon reminded, nameless people can be wonderful people.

Explaining the situation, and that it really was a matter of life and death, I said I really needed to speak with the head of Blue Cross Blue Shield, right away. She asked for a number at which I could be reached, and said she would do her best. I knew she was sincere, but I was surprised when I received a call from a physician who was either the head of the company or the head of medical review—I forget. He said he had been involved in making this decision. We had a somewhat testy discussion at first. He resented being told that his decision could be responsible for my wife's death and said that he considered the proposed surgery to be experimental. I tried not to shout and pointed out that his company had already fully approved the surgery for Dallas, Texas, and that we also had received notice that it was approved in Worcester. I also pointed out what this meant emotionally to Joan and me, after she had prepared herself to go through this frightening surgery on Monday. To his and his company's credit, he paused and said he would approve it. He didn't think the surgery should have been approved initially, but he agreed that we should not have been notified at the last minute. He arranged for a colleague to return to the office that night and fax a letter to Dr. Swanson saying the surgery would be fully financed. His colleague called me from the office, saying the letter would go out and that she would be pleased to be of assistance if other problems arise. Other, relatively small reimbursement problems did arise during the next year. She was good to her word.

Opium in the Thanksgiving Basket

We decided to celebrate Thanksgiving 1999 in Massachusetts with close friends. Joan was in the midst of a difficult course of chemotherapy. Following infusion at Sloan, we drove with the kids to Massachusetts. Joan was very nauseous and experiencing diarrhea, a problem that continued for several days. The evening before Thanksgiving she was weak and unable to eat much. Concerned that she was getting dehydrated, I called the on-call doc at Sloan, asking if we could get a prescription for tincture of opium, a drug that sometimes controls persistent diarrhea. She agreed and said she would phone it in to a pharmacy if I would get her a number. Calling the only community hospital in the area, I was put through to the hospital pharmacy. I asked whether we could purchase the drug from the hospital. The pharmacist explained that he couldn't do this but recommended that I call one of two all-night pharmacies in the region. One was not open. The other did not have tincture of opium.

I called the pharmacist back, asking if there were any way he might be able to fill the prescription. He wanted to do so, but it was against the law for a hospital pharmacy to dispense a drug—especially a highly controlled narcotic—to someone who isn't a patient. Then he thought of a way to get around this. If the on-call doc at Sloan called him, confirming the need for Joan to have the drug, perhaps Joan could be entered as a phantom patient through the emergency room. They spoke and decided an exception could be made because Joan was too ill to travel and there was no other way for her to get the medicine.

Around midnight I drove to the ER accompanied by Johanna. There I explained the situation to the intake nurse. She relayed the information to the ER doctor. Johanna and I waited. The nurse called me in to tell me that the doctor thought I would be bringing Joan to the ER. There was no way he could prescribe the drug for her without her present. But it was

Thanksgiving and I was dealing with truly concerned health care providers. She had an idea. Maybe . . . She went off to see the doc.

A few minutes later, she was admitting me as an ER patient. After taking my temperature, pulse, and blood pressure and asking me what was wrong, they prescribed tincture of opium and arranged for the pharmacy to fill it.

Johanna and I returned to our friend's home around 1:00 A.M. I woke Joan. She took the medication and went back to sleep. Thanksgiving 1999 turned into a good day. Joan felt better, and we had an enjoyable dinner with our friends.

COURAGE

It takes courage to go through cancer treatments as Joan did. It also takes courage to maintain and forge new bonds of friendship with someone diagnosed with a terminal illness, to be open to getting to know fellow patients with similar diagnoses, or for health professionals to see patients as people with families, hopes, and skills. After all, in opening yourself up to these types of relationships, you are inviting a lot of pain.

Old Friends and Family

With rare exceptions, our family, old friends, and past acquaintances did not turn away from the pain, anxiety, and discomforts of staying connected to someone who is very ill. Some, like Cathy and George, are present in nearly every chapter of this book because they were with us—either in person or conversation—at every juncture. They were there for every disappointment and for every joy. Cathy, who never did, and still doesn't, like high-tech health care settings or western medicine's sometimes obsessive and mechanical pursuit of life at all costs, took weeks of time off to help Joan, our kids, and me through this journey. Finding time to be with us was difficult; more so, finding the heart to stand by Joan's pain. George went to extraordinary lengths to help us identify and think through treatment choices, to counsel me to take care of myself, and to be a sympathetic ear. Sibling families—Dennis,

JoEllen, and Peter; Mary Jo, Scott, and Michael; Steve and Sophie and Matthew—Aunt Beth, and some cousins on both sides stayed in close touch. Friends visited from out of town. Many others kept in contact in other ways, helping to keep spirits alive and helping Joan find meaning in the days she had.

Bill Blackton

Bill was the most courageous person Joan and I knew. A friend of mine since fifth grade and Johanna's godfather, he had become very close to all of us—in some ways the sixth member of our nuclear family, Cathy being the fifth.

As kids, Bill and I would hold contests about how far we could fly paper planes from the upper-story windows of our apartment buildings. In high school, we played on the same soccer team, he passing me the ball that led to a last-minute overtime win in the league championship game. We shared the quintessential boyhood experience of being carried off the field on the shoulders of teammates. Always modest and self-effacing, Bill was liked and respected by everyone. Tenacious and kind and full of quiet humor, he was also brilliant.

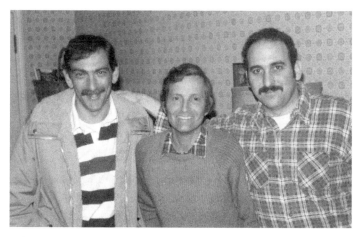

Lifelong friends George Igel, Bill Blackton, and Eric Kingson, 1985.

After graduating first in our class with perfect College Board scores, Bill had to leave Swarthmore College at the end of his first year when his kidneys failed, the result of hereditary nephritis. I recall being told by my mother that Bill was at Roosevelt Hospital in New York City and would probably not live more than a few weeks. Fortunately, Bill was selected for a kidney dialysis trial. When he died thirty-five years later, I believe he was the longest living dialysis patient in the world. He had been married twice, helped organize a national advocacy group for people with kidney diseases, worked as a news and broadcast journalist, lived in New York City, Los Angeles, and Washington, D.C., and been friend to many. Beginning in 1988, after he had a six-month hospitalization, many of our high school friends (including George Igel) participated in an event—"the Billy Bowl"—held annually in his honor. Bill would schedule us for a softball game against some similarly extraordinary athletes, before and after which there were usually marathon poker games—a lucrative sporting event from the vantage point of Bill, who was something of a card shark.

Bill had been through more than 4,000 dialysis treatments and scores of surgeries, including two failed kidney transplants. His body was crippled by arthritis and other problems related to long-term dialysis. Though in his mid-fifties, he looked more like a frail seventy-five-year-old. Still, he continued to work on the Voice of America's Mideast desk for many years, only retiring on disability a year before he died. Here, too, he was loved, so much so that his colleagues donated over one year's worth of sick leave and vacation time to enable him to receive pay during the years in which he was experiencing an increasing number of hospitalizations and disabilities.

Bill stayed in close touch with us throughout Joan's illness, up until the time he died in October 2000. Joan greatly respected Bill's desire to live and capacity to maintain humor.

Bill was in considerable pain throughout this time, and obviously failing. There was little reason to think that his body could hold on much longer. Two people who know they probably will not live as long as most have a special bond. Joan and Bill talked once a month, mostly about Johanna and Aaron but also about how Joan and Bill were doing. Joan drew strength from Bill. So when Bill commented that "Joan is a source of inspiration," I could only respond, "Bill, if she's an inspiration for you, then Joan and I must be in some really deep shit!"

Syracuse Friends and Neighbors: "Where's 'Yoan?' "

Having just moved to Syracuse, we didn't know many people there when Joan was first diagnosed. An old friend from graduate school who helped recruit me to Syracuse, Alejandro Garcia, though at first a little awkward in the face of the immensity of what was before our family, gave in ways too numerous to chronicle. A warm and gregarious spirit and a very accomplished professor, he showers friends with gifts, but none so good as the sincerity of his concern. Present at most of our family holidays, he made himself available in many ways. He brought CDs and a CD player to Joan while she was in Crouse Hospital recovering from her first surgery, gifts that got us much more involved with music than we had been. When I was put out of commission by a kidney stone attack, Aaron drove Joan to New York City for chemotherapy and Alejandro stayed at our home to watch over me. Joan was failing while Alejandro was on leave to teach in Syracuse University's London program during the spring 2001 semester. Nonetheless, he stayed in close contact with frequent e-mails and weekly calls to our home.

Faith and Jonathan Ball were new friends, a couple we had begun to form a friendship with prior to moving to Syracuse. Not wanting to be defined by her cancer, Joan took some pleasure in knowing that the roots of our friendship preceded it. Jonathan is a friend of Alejandro's, and the son of someone I consider a friend and mentor, Robert Ball—a major figure in the world of social security. Knowing I was interviewing for a position at Syracuse, Bob and his wife, Doris, suggested that Joan and I might enjoy meeting Faith and Jonathan. We did and a four-way friendship took hold. A year later, when I was offered a position at Syracuse for the second time, we got into quick contact with them. Faith, a teacher at our children's high school, gave us advice about area schools, and later about navigating Manlius High School and teenage angst in

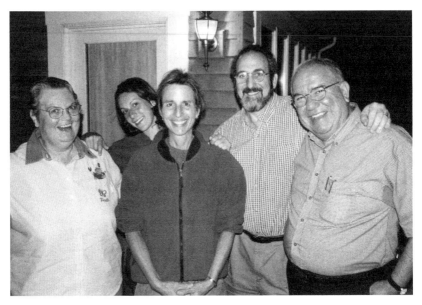

Joan's birthday celebration, September 1, 2000. Mary Bracker, Johanna, Joan, Eric, and Alejandro Garcia. Photograph courtesy of Alejandro Garcia.

suburbia. A year after Joan died, I commented to them how I thought it took courage to become friends with us. "No," Faith replied, "I didn't really think about Joan having cancer. She was so vibrant and interesting to be around. I just valued whatever time we could have." Mostly we had fun with them, and Joan enjoyed hearing stories about their young grandchildren. Just as our friends Howie and Madelyn Baum were able to celebrate the births of Aaron and Johanna when they were in the midst of their own fertility crises, Joan enjoyed hearing about the latest exploits of Faith and Jonathan's grandchildren. Sadness and tears flowed more than once about not being alive to see our grandchildren, but it was not an embittering sadness.

We had many pleasant times with Faith and Jonathan. It was a pretty regular friendship. They also served as slightly older guideposts as we navigated through life with two teenagers under new and unusual circumstances—dispensing, in response to our requests, advice on setting limits, prom etiquette, driving, and more. When we needed someone to look in on the kids or transport one of them, they made themselves easily available. And just before Joan died, it was Jonathan whom we asked to videotape Joan's messages to family members.

From the first phone call, Joe Greenman was more than the lawyer we would use to represent us to buy our Manlius house and prepare our wills. Joe's daughter Jen was in Johanna's grade and played soccer. "Yes, there's a summer team and Johanna might be able to join. I'll get you the number." Joe's wife is a school nurse. Shortly after moving, we were invited to their home. Later they gave us advice on medical practices. We took their advice. We were invited to their home in September 1998 to break the Yom Kippur fast—truthfully, we had not observed it. Not feeling well, Joan sent Aaron, Johanna, and me off by ourselves. When Joan was referred to Mark Kasowitz, we called the Greenmans. Yes, Mark was a friend and is a great doctor, if you need that kind of doc. He's scoped me and just about everyone around here. Again, good advice.

So it went with the Greenmans. Positive and open, they were a one-family information and referral service. And we enjoyed good times with them and their two children, Jen and David. They, too, gave expression to seeing a remarkable person in Joan, not her cancer.

Our neighbors Andy and Eileen Lux and their children, Sarah, Kevin, and later Mary, played a very special role in our lives and, by being themselves, brought much pleasure to Joan (and me too). Joan also brought much to them, especially the children.

Given the differences in ages between our kids and theirs, it was not foreordained that our families would get to know each other in more than a casual neighborly way. And given Joan's illness, it would have been understandable if Andy and Eileen had sought to shield their children from risking getting to know and care about someone with a terminal illness. But to their credit and our benefit, no false walls were put up. Joan, as she had done so many times before with neighbors, struck up a friendship with Eileen. Eileen's and Andy's children became regular visitors to our home, their paintings adorning our refrigerator. Joan communicated love and respect to children, and this was returned by Sarah and Kevin who were, respectively, six and three years old when we moved in. They would come by for snacks, to be read to by Joan, to play games in our basement. I would return home and often hear stories from Joan about walks and talks with them, and sometimes with Eileen. We would watch Andy in his regular after-work backyard play with Sarah and Kevin. And when Joan and I had to be away, Eileen and Andy kept an eye on our kids, Eileen always being sure they did not starve.

Later, when Mary was born, Joan delighted in watching her grow. Eileen reports, and I believe, that Mary's first word was "Joan" or, as Mary pronounced it, "Yoan." Later, when Mary reached early toddler age, she would wander—often unclothed—onto our porch, look up with her big eyes, and ask, to Joan's and my delight, "Where's Yoan?"

Three years after Joan died, Sarah, in a seventh-grade English essay, explored the feelings surrounding her last visit with Joan:

I was reading on the couch when I got the news. I don't know why I was so surprised, but I guess I just didn't expect it. She

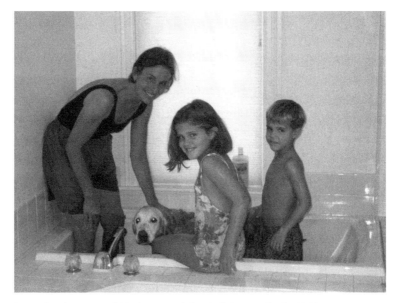

Joan, Sarah Lux, and Kevin Lux giving Baltimore a bath, 2000.

had cancer for two years now but I always thought that she would make it through.

It seemed just like yesterday that Joan and I were taking a walk at Green Lakes with her dog Baltimore. Running through the leaves and passing a ball around . . .

Over the past three months, though, I hadn't seen much of Joan. My mother told me that she wasn't feeling too good right now and tomorrow she might be feeling better, but days went by and days turned into weeks and weeks into months. Finally I had my chance; my mom had gone out to the store to get something and I was left with my dad. I decided to go over by myself for a while. As I walked over, I felt strange. I had never felt scared to go over to her house but here was a rattling in my boots. I knocked on the door and I heard a weak voice call, "Come in." As I went in I saw her. Wrapped in thin blankets with almost no shape at all with a bandanna wrapped around her head, lying in her chair helpless. I decided to sit down and tell her everything. I talked about all sorts of things. I talked about how school was going and how my friends were. I talked about my family too. Pretty soon it was dark outside and I decided to go home. "Bye" she said as I left, "Thank you for coming."

"Bye!" I said.

That was the last time I ever saw Joan and now I realize that my mother probably didn't want me to see Joan because she didn't want my last memory of her to be a bad one, and in a way it isn't. I don't remember how she looked. I just remember the ways she smiled at me in a way that said, "Everything is going to be all right."

Like the Luxes, there were many others who saw an interesting person to get to know, not a cancer patient who was dying. Sandy Lane and Cara Steinberg hired Joan as a consultant for two small projects: a study of language barriers to prenatal care for non-English-speaking women and a smoking cessation study. As always, Joan did a fine job. The willingness of Sandy and Cara to take the risk of hiring someone they knew had a stage IV diagnosis was a gift to Joan. One colleague, Deb Monahan, went out of her way to join Joan in walks at Green Lakes. Two social work graduate students, Deb Livingston and Marla Velky, and my colleague Rachael Gazdick sometimes stayed with Aaron and Johanna when Joan and I needed to travel for medical treatment. Another colleague, Bruce Lagay and his wife Helen Murray—whom we had met years ago in Australia—became fast friends. Keith Alford, whose wife, Lisa, had just given birth to a premature baby, Caleb, who required twenty-four-hour care for several years, formed a close bond with Joan. Keith, who lives nearby, brought a couple meals to us. Joan, in turn, would bring her pumpkin bread to Keith. In some undefined way, Joan and Caleb's lives seemed linked. And if Joan had to make a choice between her own and Caleb's, I have no doubt she would have chosen to breathe her life into this now six-year-old, and increasingly healthy, young child.

Our Children's Friends: Old and New

Seventeen-year-old young men are not known for their sensitivity and openness to feelings. But I recall the strength Brian Pilcher showed in allowing me to see the tears that streamed down the side of his face when I told him that Joan was extremely ill. Aaron's ebullient friend Ken Gyamfi, another seventeen-year-old, joined us in the Adirondacks, wanting as much to see Joan as to take a few days vacation. And Aaron would talk at length with Mark Citrone, whose family has also experienced more health crises than they would like, and John Simms, who had his own close brush with death.

Johanna's friends were very present: The phone lines from our home to Deirdre Salsich's and Maria Wolman's homes in Natick were in use almost daily, allowing Johanna an important intimacy and outlet with two friends who shared her love of Joan. Cards and calls from Jenna, Missy, Lily, and others gave teenage expression from Natick of concern for Johanna, Joan, and our family. New friends—Elena Toss, Emily and Megan Dutch, Jen Greenman, Samantha Karp, Carolyn Keleher, Sarah Lowenstein, and others—made themselves comfortable in our home and with Joan, again, an indication of strength of character among these young women.

Friends You Never Wanted to Meet—At Least Not This Way

Along the way, we got to know some people fairly well whose lives also had been touched by cancer. Advanced cancer is like a club—a club you do not want to join! Membership provides those with stage IV cancer, and those who are close to them, with choices that most others do not have to face so explicitly. It forces people to look deep into themselves and their relationships. The lucky ones—and they are many more than you would think—find the courage and humanity to live, laugh, cry, and continue to develop as caring human beings.

There was Barry Kearns whom I previously talked about meeting in the waiting room at Sloan. Funny and irreverent, Barry's antics kept us laughing. The circular file was his solution to managed care and bills unpaid. "What are they going to do, take my pump out? If I can get back to work, I'll pay back as much as I can. But, until then, I'm not going to worry." Once, as Joan was receiving chemotherapy, we heard laughs and giggles. A nurse was placing an IV line into Barry's arm. "Oh, yes, I like the way you do it." Nurses walked by laughing. But there was also a very serious and comforting side to Barry. When Joan, terrified of the prospect of having a pump placed in her abdomen, first asked Barry about his, he helped allay her fears. Newly married and in his mid-thirties when he was diagnosed, he hoped for a full life with his lovely wife, Olivia. But he also knew that it was up to "The Big Guy" to decide, and he would live as well as he could and trust in God.

We didn't get to know Ronnie Kasowitz, our gastroenterologist's wife, very well, but Joan valued the conversations they shared while receiving chemotherapy at Hematology-Oncology. Ronnie kept living well, just as Joan would do. And there were others. A woman with recurrent breast cancer who just kept going, and sometimes walked at Green Lakes with Joan. Joan cheered her and she Joan. When I ran into her at Green Lakes one year after Joan died, she was shocked to hear the news. "She seemed so strong. I didn't expect to hear this. Just thought she was busy."

Shortly after surgery, Joan was asked several times whether she would be willing to talk with someone who was considering similar treatments at Sloan. Joe Greenman let us know that Doug Mapstone, his client and our electrician, had just been diagnosed with pancreatic cancer and was considering surgery with Dr. Fong. A colleague at Syracuse University knew someone who was about to have the same surgery and follow-up treatment as Joan. Yet another colleague, Susan Taylor-Brown, told me her cousin Peter Goodnough had been diagnosed with sixteen liver metastases and was in very rough shape. We got to know and respect each of these people and their spouses. We shared what we had learned from Joan's prior start on the cancer path. And this giving was repaid in many ways.

Knowing Joan was having a difficult time with chemo, one day Hanna, a fellow Sloan-Kettering patient and then about seventy years old, marched into our home with a thirty-two-ounce plastic soda bottle filled with tea—marijuana tea. "Can't tell you how I got this, but it's been helpful to me and thought you might want to try it." The gift was appreciated, but Joan—having had a bad experience with marijuana in college—did not use it. Through chemo and other surgeries, Hanna has held her cancer at bay. She and her husband traveled to Brazil one week after lung surgery a few years ago. I ran into them about a couple of years ago at Syracuse's art museum. She was living well. More recently, I learned she is cancer free.

The Mapstone family went through a hellish ride. Diagnosed with pancreatic cancer, it first appeared that there was little that Doug could do and little chance of living more than a few months. We saw Doug Mapstone at Sloan, scared and depressed, after Dr. Fong determined in exploratory surgery that his tumor was not operable. With two teenage children and a marriage to his childhood sweetheart, Debbie, Doug—who ran his own electrical and plumbing business—fought through chemotherapies to buy good, but also often painful time. Joan, Debbie, Debbie's mom, Doug, and I kept in touch by telephone, each giving support to the other. Joan was not well enough to attend Doug's funeral, so I went for both of us. When Joan died a few months later, Debbie and her mother—raw from their grief—attended Joan's funeral.

We first spoke with Peter and Nancy Goodnough by telephone after Peter had made the decision to have surgery with Dr. Fong. "I'm a realist," Peter probably communicated. "I know the score. I have multiple metastases, a couple of which may not be operable; I am hoping to buy some good time." One of Joan's appointments with Dr. Kemeny coincided with Peter's surgery, so we were able to meet Nancy and one of her daughters while she waited to hear news of the surgery. A day later we met Peter, in good humor, in his hospital room. "Fong took out fourteen mets and fried the two that were not resectable" (that is, used radio frequency ablation). As Peter, a surgeon, put it, "that took guts." He was delighted with the outcome. He was able to return to his own surgical practice in Cooperstown, New York, and to make good use of much of the time that was left.

Joan and Peter formed a fast and lasting bond. Peter, like Joan, was an avid reader. A spiritual and religious man, he was not afraid to think about his death. He and Joan provided support and humor to each other by telephone. Not fearing death, shortly before his death, Peter asked to see the tape Joan left for our family. When I visited him and Nancy in Cooperstown, a few weeks before his death, he was visibly weak, but still engaged in reading, conversation, and poetry.

When we met Bill Fenton in the Sloan waiting room, he and his wife, Karen, had been dealing with metastatic colon cancer for about seven years. I'm not sure how the conversation started, but we were probably all finding something funny. Nancy Kemeny had previously "bombed" Bill's cancer into remission with a massive dose of chemotherapy. The remission lasted about five years, and now it had come roaring back, and he was entering the same phase II trial as Joan— CPT-11 and Oxaliplatin.

Bill, an avid golfer and retired from the insurance industry, had a home in Palm Beach County, Florida. He was great fun to argue with. Like my favorite uncle (also called "Bill"), Bill Fenton was more conservative in his politics than I. He was getting increasingly ill around the time of the Bush/Gore presidential election (who could blame him for that!!). I'm not sure he particularly liked either candidate, but he had decided to vote for Gore. I would joke with him, "Look, you can't die before the election. We need every vote." Later, when Palm Beach County was embroiled in the postelection recount, Joan and I quipped, "Bill, you can't check out before the election results are in." He didn't. He managed to play a couple more rounds of golf before dying. I remain in touch with Karen, whose humor and optimism is leading her down new paths, including that of teaching yoga to elders in Florida.

Health Care Providers

We came to recognize the commitment of many who provide health care to people with cancer as a form of courage. It is difficult to see the pain experienced by the patients and their families. More so, to see the humanity in the people you are treating, to endure the loss of patients for whom you cared. Even when there are positive outcomes—and there are many—cancer patients must often endure great discomfort and pain. The phlebotomist who searches out veins, the nurse who helps address nausea, the chaplain who comforts family, the nurse's aides who get patients up and moving after surgery, the doctors, and the nurses . . . Each is challenged every day to not depersonalize and to remember that they are dealing with people with histories, skills, and hopes. Some close off to their patients. But, as numerous examples in the book attest, many have the courage to see the humanity in the people they serve.

HUMOR

Comforting the Sick

Joan was three days past her twelve-hour surgery, and we were talking in her room, when we heard a knock. "Hello, may I come in?" asked a 140-year-old woman standing at the entrance to Joan's room.

Hearing the words "I'm the Catholic chaplain," Joan threw back her head and feigned being comatose. "May I come in?" Not wanting to get in the way of Joan and her religion of origin, I said, "Sure."

"Is this Joan Kingson's room?"

"Yes," I said.

"Do you mind if I say a prayer for your wife?"

"Thank you. I'm Jewish, but that would be very nice."

After calling upon Jesus by name to bring health to Joan, she asked if I believed Jesus could do that. I responded that I believe God manifests itself in many ways. "Yes, but do you believe that He can heal her?" I responded that I was Jewish and had different beliefs. Not missing a beat, she responded, "That's alright, the Jews are the chosen people." ("Good thing to know. Thanks for the reminder," I thought to myself.) Turning toward her, I thanked her for her prayer. Joan remained "comatose." As she was leaving the room, the chaplain turned around and said, "Oh, by the way, you don't have to feel bad about the Jews killing Christ." ("More good news," I thought. Not exactly a major preoccupation as I sat in the hospital room worrying about whether Joan would recover from her surgical ordeal, but I managed to remain cordial.) "It was the Romans who killed Christ, not the Jews." "Thanks," I replied, thinking that she must have just heard about the Vatican's statement exonerating Jews. Turning to Joan, I thanked her for providing me with this opportunity for religious education and assured her that I would cut off her oxygen supply if she ever left me alone in the room with this woman again.

Shopping for Wigs

Joan wasn't vain. She didn't use much makeup and had little patience for fashions. But after the chemo beat up her hair follicles for the third time, she tried to find a wig. At about this time, Sloan opened a small store on the top floor of its outpatient facility with specialized items for patients—what we promptly dubbed "Your Cancer Boutique." Walking through the store, listening to soothing music and looking at the selection of wigs, scarves, inspirational tapes, healing stones, and self-help books, we decided "The Shop 'Til You Drop Store" would be a more suitable name.

Our cynicism not withstanding, Joan bought two wigs—the first from a store in the Syracuse area and the second from "Shop 'Til You Drop." Neither wig ever made it onto Joan's head for more than a few minutes. The first just didn't work, not even after Joan brought it to a hairdresser known to work well with wigs. It was too coiffed for her taste. But we got our money's worth in entertainment. Johanna, Joan, and Helen Osborne, a friend from Natick who was visiting, had a hilarious time with it, trying it on, making faces and eventually deciding that it looked best on a large jar of peanut butter, sitting on the kitchen countertop. The second—and by far the more elegant wig—came to rest on the head of a stuffed toy, a monkey that was in residence on Joan's dresser.

Joan decided to wear floral scarves. She looked beautiful, and I learned to think of these scarves as badges of courage. Toward the end of her life, she shaved her head. She was more beautiful than ever. Radiant and in no need of makeup or wigs.

Upbeat Greetings at Sloan

"Hello. Come on in. Good to see you again. And how are you. Lovely to see you." The two male receptionists, John Morales and Raymond Caballero, greeted all who came to Sloan's outpatient facility with cheerful respect. Not exactly what you expect to find as you walk in for chemotherapy or presurgical consultation with your oncologist or surgeon. But their sincere friendliness and humor provided an air of levity that was appreciated by most everyone. There were exceptions, such as the woman Joan and I heard muttering under her breath, "Somebody's going to kill that guy one day."

Get Your Hands Off Me

We were sitting on plastic covered chairs in the basement of Sloan, waiting for Joan to be called for a ultrasound. Four or five other patients and family members were in the area, mostly flipping through magazines. Out of nowhere we heard a woman screaming, "Get your hands off me; I want to go home." We looked around wondering what was going on. Down the hall, we saw a woman being wheeled on a gurney accompanied by an attendant and nurse. "Get your fuckin' hands off me; I know my rights. I want to go home!" We shrugged our shoulders and smiled uncomfortably at the other people around us. More commotion. Security guards joined the nurse. "We have to bring you back to your room, Ma'am. If you still want to leave when you get there, you may." Irrational, abusive, and loud, she continued, "No, I want to go home now. I don't want to go to the room. I know my rights. Get your goddamn hands off me. I want to leave right now." Joan and I commented to each other that, by now, they must be tempted to open the door to the street and help her on her way.

A long day, Joan had chemotherapy and was feeling very peaked as we drove home to Syracuse that night. She took some Ativan and slept. As we often did, I stopped at the Liberty Diner, a good midway point, and ordered soup to go for Joan and a hot dog and coffee for me. Feeling a little better, we started to talk about the day. She commented that as crazy and obnoxious as that woman seemed, in some ways she was giving voice to what every patient at Sloan feels. No more scans, no more needle sticks, no more chemo, no more docs. We started to get giddy, envisioning patients leaving Sloan in droves. "Yeh, guys, she's right. Let's all get the hell out of here."

A month or so later, we wandered into the type of shop you find in many student areas, in this case Marshall Street near the Syracuse University campus. Browsing through the inventory that included inexpensive leather goods, crystals, hookahs, and T-shirts, I came to a black shirt with "Get the fuck away from me" emblazoned across the front. We laughed. Yes, this was the perfect shirt for Joan to wear the next time she goes to Sloan!

A few weeks later I bought the shirt as a joke. Of course, Joan never wore it. But as she was dying at Crouse Hospital, she gave it to Linda Butler and told her to give it to her fiancé, a retired undercover drug cop, who has a special way with words.

Joan's Last Words

For almost three years, I had been the cheerleader, the one looking for the next treatment and the miracle that would allow us to grow old together. But by early May 2001, the goal shifted to Joan having a good death. Just after calling an end to continued hydration and nutrition, Joan said to me, "Eric, I don't know if I am going to be able to die with you present. You bring me back." My response: "Listen, Hon, you die anyway the hell you want." She smiled. Mindful of her concern about my making it difficult for her to let go, a few days later, after she had drifted into a coma, I sat by her bed saying, "It's okay, Hon, it's time for you to go. It's time to die." Breaking through the coma for a moment, she said with a smile, "It sure as hell is, Eric!" She died two days later, in my arms, a wry smile on her face.

6

Final Months

∫℘ The last six months of Joan's life were a gift to her family and friends. And I like to think and believe they were a gift to her as well. She was very loving and very loved.

My abiding image of this period is of her sitting in our family room, on a hunter green leather chair, reclining with her feet up and a red fleece blanket covering her from the chest down. Warmed by the blanket and wood stove, she read novels, listened to the news on NPR, and remained present for family and others in our home, savoring every moment of family life, more precious with each day because at one level she and we knew.

Although weakened by two years of surgeries, chemotherapy, and cancer, she was physically active for most of this time and fully engaged with life until a few days before her death.

Afternoon or night, she was there—even when exhausted—to edit Johanna's papers, to work with Aaron on college essays, to listen to the latest story I brought home from work. Soccer dinners, track meets, school conferences. She supported Aaron's involvement at the Boys and Girls Clubs. When one of the kids Aaron recruited as a volunteer—an inner-city African American girl from Brooklyn who was living in a special community-supported residence—made a foolish mistake that almost resulted in her being sent back home to New York City, Joan, though by then quite weak, wrote a letter appealing her situation to the board of directors of the residence.

A steady stream of the kids' friends made their way to our kitchen.

Out-of-town visitors too—Cathy, Mary Jo, Dennis, Jo Ellen, Linda Butler Masters, Michele Melville, Marcia Hartley, Judy and Deirdre Salsich, Loretta and Maria Wolman, Helen Osborne, Scott and Susan Plumb, Gayle Mosher, Rob Hudson, and others.

She kept up her daily walks with Baltimore. We made plans to go away for a short vacation in early January. We hosted a Christmas party for the school of social work, something we wanted to do as a way of thanking my colleagues who had been so giving.

DECEMBER 2000–MARCH 2001

But another early-December event is more memorable. Joan was maid of honor at the marriage of a high school friend, Brigit Kennedy, near Hartford, Connecticut. We tried something new. Johanna would visit friends in Boston, and Aaron would stay in Syracuse. A seemingly model young person, we agreed to let him stay at home by himself. "Don't worry. I'll be fine." He was.

Saturday evening, the night of the wedding reception, we received a call from Aaron. "Hi Dad, just want to check in with you guys. How was the wedding? How's Mom? By the way, where are you staying tonight? You're not driving in this snowstorm?" I told him not to worry. He wasn't.

Arriving home the next day, the house was clean, too clean. A small piece of hardware had fallen off the bottom of the sectional couch. A quick look in the garbage can in the garage told the story. One of the sixty or so kids who, I later learned, had partied through the night at our house had left an empty bottle of beer in the trash. I confronted Aaron. "Aaron, I want the truth!" I got it—at least most of it (the rest coming in funny stories three and four years later). I was furious. Joan was upset, but, as was often the case, her anger more measured. She did say, though, that what Aaron had done made her uncomfortable with leaving the kids for a week, even with an adult in the house. This made me more furious. Aaron, who had been urging me to plan a trip alone with his mom—just in case she did not live much longer—had now made this impossible by his actions. There was no way Joan would leave the nest now.

Well, like many things in life that seem so bad at the time, it turned out to be for the best. After punishing Aaron and taking away his right to drive for the next sixty-five years, I canceled our vacation plans. A few weeks later, Joan and I decided that since we were not comfortable leaving the kids, we should take them with us. We bought four tickets to Puerto Rico, got terrific post-Christmas season rates for a second floor villa overlooking the ocean at the Rio Del Mar Westin Resorts, and took the kids out of school for a week.

Puerto Rico

It was a wonderful vacation, every day full of sun and warmth. Like the decision to buy our Adirondack home and to go to Australia, this was one of those experiences we were very thankful to have had as a family. It gave us time—time to all be together, time away from cancer, and time to enjoy the moment . . . Time to deny what was to come. And time, though brief, that felt like forever.

The resort absorbed the kids, especially Aaron who was fascinated by casino life. Joan and I were not "resort people." Our idea of travel was staying in modest hotels, walking through marketplaces, talking with people, eating in local restaurants and visiting museums, aquariums, and natural habitats. That's what the kids were used to. But they adapted quickly to jet skiing, tanning, and mixing with other tourists at the Westin pools. And we all enjoyed fruit-laden poolside buffet breakfasts.

Joan and I took a couple of drives—to a rain forest, to Old San Juan, and to some small towns and villages. But mostly we enjoyed the kids, the quiet pleasure of walking by the sea, and sitting on the terrace of our two-room villa. Joan was relaxed even though she was experiencing some pulls in her abdomen from the tumors. We would walk a couple hundred yards, and then she might bend over for twenty seconds or so to take pressure off the tumors. I slowed my pace—a first in our twenty-three years of being together. No complaints from her; just acknowledgment that these things must be growing. We would deal with them with

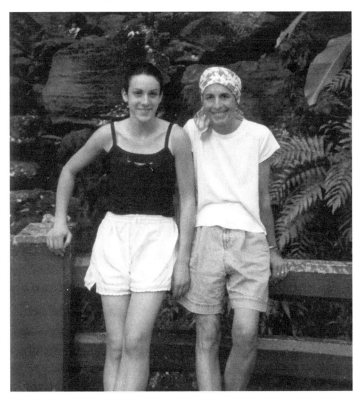

Johanna and Joan in Puerto Rico, January 2001.

a new approach to chemo that would begin at the end of January—we thought, we hoped. We picked up shells, greeted people who passed by, and I proudly held the hand of the woman I loved and so respected as we walked, talked, and laughed through the week.

After Puerto Rico, Joan's health went downhill, slowly through mid-March and then rapidly. We maintained a hope that we could still buy many years but not the expectation.

At the beginning of the cancer treatments, Joan was clear that she did not want treatments to undermine her quality of life. Over time, her assessment of trade-offs and definition of "quality" changed. In spite of the discomforts of chemo, pump, ileostomy, needle sticks, exhaustion, and various gastric unpleasantries, she was still enjoying living, family,

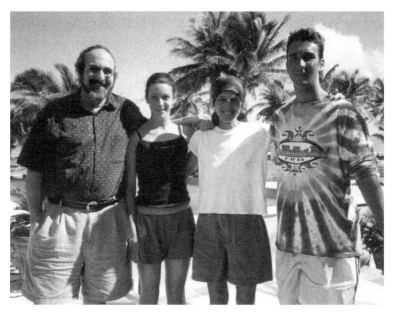

"Timeless" time in Puerto Rico: Eric, Johanna, Joan, and Aaron, January 2001.

friends, pets, and novels. She didn't fear death but was not ready to greet it as a release. If we could buy more time, this would be good.

Seeking Access to a "Wonder Drug"

Beginning in late October 2000, Dr. Kemeny and Dr. Scalzo had started Joan on another chemo regimen, administered mostly in Syracuse. With their approval, George and I strategized about gaining access to C-225 (now called Erbitux), a promising monoclonal antibody. Dr. Kemeny and Dr. Scalzo thought it worth a try. The hope was that the chemo cocktail Joan was getting would at a minimum buy enough time until we could gain access to C-225 or something else.

Preliminary results from C-225 trials were very promising. Twenty-two percent of persons with highly treated metastatic colon cancer whose tumors were receptive to epidermal growth factors (EGF positive) showed marked reductions in tumors or remissions when treated with this drug. Joan's tumor cells had been tested in October 1999 by Imclone, the company pioneering C-225. The results suggested that this new drug might be beneficial. Given what we were dealing with, it was the best hope in town.

While we still explored other interventions, we pinned a lot of our hope on getting this drug under compassionate-use protocol. We had been placed on the company's waiting list, but that was a while ago and we did not need the drug until now—Joan had been responding to the other treatments available. I called the company's research office and spoke with the physician in charge of the compassionate-use program. Yes, he understood that Joan had been tested by the company and that she once was on the waiting list. However, with all the publicity the drug was getting, the company had closed the waiting list, and there was nothing he could do. There was a very limited supply of the drug, held mainly for clinical trials the company was sponsoring. "Couldn't you simply reinstate her on the basis that she was once on the list?" "No," he replied. I asked if there was any way to get the drug through the National Cancer Institute or anywhere else. "No." Merck KGA, a German drug company, had bought the right to distribute the drug in European trials, and I had learned that they had on occasion made it available outside the trials. "Could you give me the name of your parallel in Merck KGA? I'd like to see if maybe we could get C-225 outside the country." "No."

I learned that the Federal Drug Administration (FDA) had raised some questions about what the agency considered Imclone's overly liberal release of the drug for compassionate use, possibly a backdoor vehicle for getting the drug into circulation. The company seemed to be battening down the hatches.

At my request, a close friend called on behalf of a U.S. senator, indicating the senator's concern and asking if a direct contact from the senator might make a difference. The doctor wouldn't budge. He indicated that there simply was not enough supply, and if Joan was given the drug, it would mean not giving it to someone else who was already on the priority list.

A couple months passed, and the cancer was advancing in Joan's liver. Dr. Kemeny reactivated Joan's liver pump, hoping that delivering chemo directly would hold off the cancer.

I learned that Imclone was expanding its production of C-225. Another round of calls to the physician heading Imclone's compassionate-use program was getting us nowhere. Advised by a couple of people that Dr. Harlan Waksal—then Imclone's medical director, brother of its CEO, and the boss of the compassionate-use gatekeeper—was a decent and empathetic person, I sent a direct appeal to him in January. I had previously spoken with his secretary, who seemed sympathetic to our situation, and sensed that she would pass a letter on to her boss. Putting our best foot forward, I described our family, Joan's situation and the basis of our appeal (see letter in appendix B). Following up the letter with a telephone call, Dr. Waksal's secretary passed me directly to her boss. Yes, he had read the letter. I explained the situation again, including the discussions that had taken place with the physician in charge of the compassionate-use program. Dr. Waksal offered to look into the situation and said that he would also ask that the waiting list be reviewed.

He was good to his word. In February, Dr. Waksal got back to me and said that because Imclone had documentation of our May 2000 telephone call, Joan had been reinstated on the waiting list and she was now approved to receive C-225 (see appendix B for my notes on this telephone call). There were still some details to work out, but it looked as if Joan would be able to start the drug in a few weeks. I was ecstatic and deeply appreciative.

Imclone has since been rocked by insider trading scandals. The company was the subject of congressional hearings similar to the Enron and Global Crossings hearings. Harlan's brother, Sam Waksal, was forced to resign as CEO and later convicted of insider trading. He is now serving time in a federal penitentiary. Martha Stewart, a friend of Sam Waksal, was similarly convicted of insider trading. The Federal Drug Administration (FDA) rejected Imclone's December 2001 bid for approval of C-225, or Erbitux, on the grounds that the clinical trial sampling was faulty. Results from a 2003 study by a German company with the European rights to the drug seem to have confirmed Imclone's earlier findings that the drug is effective.

Two-and-one-half years after Joan died, on February 12, 2004, Imclone issued a press release indicating Erbitux's status:

ImClone Systems Incorporated (Nasdaq: IMCL) and Bristol-Myers Squibb Company (NYSE: BMY) announced today that the U.S. Food and Drug Administration (FDA) has approved ERBITUX(TM) (Cetuximab) Injection for use in combination with Ironetecan in the treatment of patients with EGFR-expressing, metastatic colorectal cancer who are refractory to Ironetecan-based chemotherapy and for use as a single agent in the treatment of patients with EGFR-expressing, metastatic colorectal cancer who are intolerant to Ironetecan-based chemotherapy.

In other words, the drug is now approved by the FDA for use with people in Joan's situation.

MARCH–MAY 2001

Final Weeks at Home

It was a very difficult time. Yet, in ways I cannot fully explain, it was also a wonderful time because there was no doubt in our home and hearts that we were all deeply committed to each other. Her humor intact, Joan still found family, friends, pets, and reading pleasurable—maybe especially so because she understood the likely choices and changes in front of us. In January, when Aaron received an "Unsung Hero's Award" for his volunteer work, Joan and I had proudly attended Syracuse University's annual Martin Luther King dinner and ceremony, beaming with parental pride. She was weak then but still able to get around. By March, she was unable to attend the ceremony where Aaron was installed as Syracuse's youth of the year. I wrote to friends:

Aaron continues to have a wonderful senior year, in all ways, except of course Joan's health. He's become a confident young man and has a good social life. He has spent much of his time during this year building a volunteer program that involves about eighty kids from his high school in volunteer work at a Boys and Girls Club. My friend and colleague, Alejandro Garcia, nominated Aaron for an unsung hero award that he received in the annual Syracuse Martin Luther King event, keynoted by Cornell West. A few weeks later Aaron also was named Syracuse "Youth of the Year." Of course we're very proud, but do you have any idea how tough it is to live with the "Youth of the Year!" Imagine trying to discipline him. "But Dad . . ." Worse yet, he is being considered for "Youth of the Year" for New York State! About a month ago, Aaron was hired as half-time coordinator of volunteers for the Boys and Girls Clubs of Syracuse. His involvement with the clubs is a real passion for him, so much so that he gave up playing tennis this spring. College? Looks as if he will be going to Syracuse University and working at the Boys and Girls Clubs while majoring in economics and possibly public policy. He may visit a couple of the other schools that accepted him (GWU, University of Rochester, and William and Mary) but it is likely that he will choose SU. I have to admit that Joan and I would like to see him remain close to us.

Johanna is equally wonderful, though life has been a little less eventful for her, even though she is no less eventful for us. Her circle of friends is growing and deepening. She and they have good taste in friends. She is kind and insightful and full of energy and fun. She continues to work hard and do exceptionally well in school. Rather than run spring track, she decided to learn a new sport and has become a member of the JV lacrosse team. She's loving it, only we wish she wouldn't play it so much in our house. Joan's illness is hard on all of us, but right now we worry most about Johanna as she is younger, and it feels to us a little more vulnerable. But we also have confidence that she and Aaron are handling the challenges it brings in constructive ways.

Joan's health had been going downhill rapidly. She had been greatly weakened by the cancer and the chemotherapies. From January forward, Joan had difficulty keeping food down. She now needed help in and out of the bathtub. Diarrhea was chronic. Eating had become more difficult, both because of the nausea that often followed chemotherapy (with CPT-11) and, as we would later learn, because an abdominal tumor was blocking the exit from her stomach. She lost weight and strength.

To prevent dehydration, Dr. Scalzo and Dr. Kemeny started home infusions, two liters a day in a backpack so she could move around if she wished. We were trained in its use, and again, adjusted to the presence of this new equipment in our lives. A few weeks later, Joan began intravenous nutrition.

We, and especially Joan, knew that she was not going to be able to live much longer, but we were still hoping that we might gain access to C-225 or another treatment that would buy good time. It took a while to work out some of the administrative issues, but C-225 was delivered to Dr. Scalzo's office under a compassionate-use agreement. Joan was scheduled to start chemo infusion with the drug at Dr. Scalzo's office on April 12. It was looking as if this was none too soon. Joan had pretty much decided that this was the last treatment she would try.

Joan was getting sicker and more uncomfortable by the day, unable to hold food and liquids and finding it increasingly difficult to negotiate the stairs and bathtub. Still she would sit and read and remain available to close family and friends. April 9, 10, and 11 were particularly bad days. And on the eleventh, Joan and I agreed that she was too weak to stay at home. She didn't like the idea of another hospitalization but agreed that it was necessary. I didn't like the idea either because I was afraid it might derail the C-225 treatment, but it seemed cruel for her to remain at home. I called Dr. Scalzo's office, and he arranged for her to be admitted to Crouse Hospital. A few days to regain her strength, we hoped, and then we could start treatment.

Settling in to Room 4005

We moved into room 4005 on the fourth floor of Crouse Hospital. The lease expired on May 12.

Terry Principato, the nurse-practitioner on the oncology floor, helped settle us into the room. IVs started. A comforting directness, combined with a sense of caring competence. Words of reassurance. Yes, the goal was to stabilize Joan, and then get her back home as soon as possible. Yes, they would get me a reclining chair on which I could sleep, but I was told I may be more comfortable sleeping on the empty bed. (Now there's an idea!)

A quick visit from Warren Hughes, an outgoing nurse's aide, who always had a kind word, a witty comment, and often a gift for patients. There is a depth to his compassion and commitment to helping people. Good medicine often manifests itself best through smiles and gentle kindnesses freely dispensed.

Soon we had little doubt about the wisdom of this admission to the hospital. With some luck, we would be out in a couple of days.

The next day's tests revealed that Joan's tumor was blocking the passage of food from her stomach. No surprise now why eating had become so difficult and ineffective. A decision was made to place a tube (called a peg tube) in her stomach to make her more comfortable.

As I recall, Dr. Scalzo was out of town. One of his partners, Dr. Richard Cherney was standing in for him. A gentle and spiritual man, he forged a close and quick connection with Joan. When we met, I explained our concern to start C-225 as soon as possible. I indicated that the permission we received allowed for its use in any way Dr. Scalzo or Dr. Kemeny wished. We discussed the possibility of starting the treatment in the hospital. Recognizing that we were in an uphill battle with time, within a couple of days he would act on this information.

The medicine arrived on Friday morning, before the peg tube was inserted. While Joan was waiting for this minor surgery, Terry came into

Joan's room and said that they were ready to set up an IV for a test run of C-225. Assuming it went well (which it did), they would start the full infusion as soon as Joan returned from the OR.

No negative response—Joan was ready to start this new chemo. But first she was brought down to the OR. The procedure went well, but when she returned to the room, there was more bleeding than anticipated. Somewhat crestfallen, we all agreed to hold off starting the treatment until Monday.

The bleeding stopped. The weekend passed uneventfully. Visits from Aaron, Johanna, and friends; cards, paintings from the Lux children; lots of cards and little gifts. Pictures, children's paintings, and cards went up on the wall. We decorated the room with stuffed animals, most notably one of Johanna's monkeys hanging from the ceiling.

No one had been admitted to fill the vacant bed in Joan's room yet, and so I had a fairly comfortable place to sleep at night. No matter how good the hospital care, there is no substitute for having a caring, loving family member or friend around. Hospitals are terribly busy places, and nursing and housekeeping staffs are under tremendous pressure. I was happily at Joan's "beck and call"—running errands to get more water, straws to drink chicken broth, new sheets, extra pillows, and so forth. I was there to help her shower, to help her move from bed to toilet, to take—when she still could—a few very short walks. I was also there to keep an eye on the medications; to be sure that Joan was getting what she needed when she needed it. And, when Joan's stomach tube was plugged, I was—thanks to the instruction of one of the physicians— there to drain it, something I probably did at least ten times a day.

But mostly, I was company for Joan. I was there to love and hold her hand; to try to keep her spirits up, and mine, too; to step aside when special family and friends were with her. We laughed a lot, cried, and just were.

Of course I still had a job. The semester was still progressing, and I continued to meet my classes; correct papers, and do my best to fulfill obligations at school. After a few days, Cathy came up from Boston to take care of the home front. She stayed with the kids and visited with

Joan during the day. At night, sitting outside Joan's room, I would read student papers while Joan slept. It was a surrealistic experience, but one that I treasure. But I have gotten a bit ahead of myself.

Easter Magic

Easter weekend passed pleasantly. Lots of visitors, laughter, and quiet times together. On Easter Sunday I gave a magic show for the few kids who remained on the hospital's pediatric floor. Joan and I were grateful for the care she was receiving, and performing magic for kids seemed like a small way to pay back the hospital and put smiles on the faces of a few kids. "If I am really good," I may have thought, "Maybe God will . . . ?"

Johanna helped me to set up some of the props. Sue Karl, then the child life specialist at Crouse, introduced herself. We talked about Joan, who she knew by reputation to be one of the leaders among child life professionals. Doing the show in the hospital was reminiscent of my first shows at Roosevelt Hospital in New York City, where I had volunteered as a sixteen-year-old in the child life department. And of the show I gave when Joan was the child life training coordinator at Johns Hopkins Hospital.

The show went well. Afterwards, I talked with some of the kids, one in particular who was very interested in learning about magic. I ended up bringing him a magic kit a couple of days later, and he, in turn, made a model plane that he gave to the "magician." This is some of the fun and reward of doing magic. But the show also led me down a path that would be very beneficial for Joan and me.

After the show, I ran into Reverend Terry Culbertson, at the time the head of Pastoral Counseling at Crouse. Guitar tucked by her side, Terry commented that the kids seemed all tired out from the magic show. I wasn't sure if that was a good or bad comment about my prestidigitation skills, but it provided an opening for Sue to introduce us and mention that Joan was in the hospital. Terry's offer to visit was gladly accepted. Unlike the pastoral representative at UMass-Worcester, Terry is neither intrusive nor insensitive to people of other faiths. Although

Terry is an evangelical minister, I would later learn that Terry's husband is Jewish and that her daughter was preparing for her bat mitzvah.

I overheard Sue and Terry talking about something called "Reiki" and a research project involving its use on pediatrics. "What is Reiki?" I asked. They explained that it was a healing technique involving the passing of energy, not too dissimilar from the nursing idea of the "healing touch." Some of the staff on the adult oncology floor had been trained in its use by Don Brennan, a local Reiki master. At worst it seemed benign. At best, I thought, there might be something to this.

Compassionate Use Awry

Monday, April 15, I left the hospital to teach my morning class of undergraduate social work students. Ironically, we were in the health policy section of the course.

I called Joan after class, expecting to hear that the C-225 infusion had begun. I was stunned to learn that Dr. Scalzo had canceled the chemotherapy.

A major bureaucratic nightmare had occurred. Imclone's director of clinical trials had called indicating that the drug could not be administered at Crouse Hospital and ordered that it be destroyed.

I called Imclone's director of clinical trials. Speaking in calm, low tones, I asked him why Joan could not start this treatment. Even though we had been told that the drug could be used in any reasonable manner, the protocol, he insisted, required that it be administered only at the Hematology-Oncology office or at St. Joseph's Hospital. He claimed that hand-carrying the drug from the Hematology-Oncology offices to Crouse Hospital had placed Hematology-Oncology's research capacity at risk. The drug might have been contaminated if it was opened by the person who transported it—as if someone was likely to break open its seal. If Hematology-Oncology didn't destroy the drug, the FDA could even press charges, he said. Some of the docs might lose their licenses. At no time did he show the slightest concern for Joan or what we were going through as a family.

Holding my anger in check, I started to say, "Dr. X, this has nothing to do with politics, just . . ." He cut me off with a sharp retort. "Are you trying to threaten me?" Again, replying in quiet tones I said, "No, Dr. X, this is just a husband who very much loves his wife and wants her to have this last chance for more life. How can we get past this to help her?" His response was astounding as it was piercing. "Well, it probably won't do her any good at this point, anyway." We talked some more, and he agreed that there was an outside chance that Imclone might be able to send out another batch of drugs once this mess got cleared up. I thanked him for keeping the option open, even though what I really wanted to do was leap through the phone and strangle him.

Reiki

I knew that the pain and discomfort of the disease had mostly overtaken Joan's interest in further treatment. She knew, better than I was willing to admit, that the chances of buying quality time were slim to none. C-225 represented the last thing she would try, in part, I think, because Joan knew how hard I had worked to gain access and how much I wanted her to have more time.

Never to be without a plan or without some hope, I began talking with some of the nurses and aids on the unit about Reiki. They were very positive about the experience. Several commented that they never saw it do any harm, and that it seemed to be helpful to a fair number of patients. One attributed her brother's survival of stage IV cancer to daily Reiki sessions she did with him when he was extremely ill. That was enough for me. Maybe this was the miracle. But more likely, maybe this was the vehicle for helping Joan to keep her spirits up and hang on long enough until we once again gained access to C-225.

I called Don Brennan, the Reiki master who had trained Terry and some of the Crouse nurses and nurse's aides. I explained the situation and my goals. We talked about Reiki. Satisfied that he seemed to be neither a charlatan or messianic "new ager," I asked him if he would be willing to help us. He didn't make any promises of miracles, and I didn't expect any (though I would have gladly accepted one). I wanted to sustain Joan and maintain hope. Indeed, we did find sustenance, but not in the way I expected.

Don came to the hospital the following day. A thin man with gentle features, he was carrying a portable CD player. We shook hands. His hands were slightly gnarled and perhaps inflamed. Some healer, I might have thought in a more cynical moment, but as I would find out, he did indeed have a healing heart and touch.

Joan decided to try this. Neither she nor I knew what to expect, but we figured she didn't have much to lose. Cathy—trained in yoga and Pilates—was open to Joan giving Reiki a try. Don, Cathy, Reverend Culbertson, a Buddhist chaplaincy trainee (who was also a Reiki master), and I participated in the Reiki session.

Don first spoke privately to Joan. He then invited the four of us into the room, and, with soft electronic music playing quietly, he instructed us on what to do and where to position ourselves around Joan. Cathy and I, new to Reiki, were told to concentrate on passing healing energy from our hands to Joan. We didn't have to touch Joan for the energy to pass, but could if Joan did not mind. We might want to concentrate on some of the chakra points. As I recall, he directed that areas on the sole, palm, arm and leg joints, and head were particularly open to receiving energy. Mainly we should try to feel the energy around Joan's body and let the Reiki flow to where it is most needed. Joan closed her eyes and tried to relax. Don and I were across from each other at the head of the bed, Cathy was next to me, and the chaplains close to Joan's feet.

Don started near Joan's head and the upper part of her torso. I looked at Joan with love and hope, letting my hands pass above her head and chest. "God, I love her. Maybe there is something to this," I thought, I hoped. I recall thinking that it seemed pretty strange to be holding what seemed one step removed from a séance in a modern hospital. Even more extraordinary, the nurses and even the physicians were treating this with respect. One of the doctors from Joan's oncology practice came into the room toward the middle of the session. Seeing five adults—including the chief chaplain—moving their hands over his patient must have looked a bit out of the ordinary to him. Respectfully, he left and returned when the session ended.

After thirty minutes or so, Don asked Joan if she was feeling anything. "Yes, it feels like heat going to the areas of my body that have the largest tumors." I was surprised. "Maybe a miracle is possible," I thought. I concentrated harder and focused even more on how much I loved Joan, and how much I wanted more time together. She seemed to drift off. Forty or fifty minutes later, she opened her eyes, simultaneously smiling and crying, releasing tears that long needed to come forth.

"I feel connected to everything. I realize I, we, are all part of something that continues." Then she started to sob, "I realize that I am worth loving, that I really deserve to be loved. This is so hard for me. I knew I am a good person. But there's always been something in me, until now, that held me back from feeling deserving and fully accepting of love. I was good at giving love, but had a harder time accepting it.

"I had this vision that I was at a warm lake in the Adirondacks. I cast off all these tubes, jumped in nude and swam to an island. I made a campfire and began waiting for everyone else to get there. This is how I see dying. I'll be there, waiting for all of you."

While very intuitive and having a sense of connection to a larger force for good in the universe, visions and giving expression to religious/spiritual beliefs was not characteristic of Joan. Only in childbirth had I ever seen Joan display such intensity of spiritual emotion. I was pleased and hopeful. I'll confess that beyond the love I felt for Joan, I could not feel energy fields or flows from me to her. But my mind was open, and I was relieved when Cathy said that she had felt the energy around Joan.

Don arranged to return in a couple of days. We held another session, involving Cathy, Johanna, and several close friends. This, too, was intense, but less than the first session. It was interrupted a number of times by the need to flush Joan's peg tube. Joan reported having a vision of being reincarnated as a porpoise and swimming in the ocean. Joan's friend Linda laughed because she too was thinking about water and swimming among fish. The session was shorter because of Joan's discomfort.

Afterwards, while Joan rested, Don instructed Cathy and me in Reiki. During the weeks to come, I would spend a little time each day, often while Joan slept, trying magically to improve her health. At times, one of the nurse's aides would do so as well.

As I have experimented with some of what Don taught me, I have satisfied myself that there is much of value in Reiki. Most startling, from my point of view, was my discovery that I can run my fingertips near the palm of many people's hands in a way that enables most to feel energy from me even though we are not touching. This knowledge/experience is a source of hope. Perhaps much of what we are is "just" energy. I like to think that perhaps, when we die, our energy joins with that of others we love. I hope so.

Living amid Her Good-Byes

While skeptical about whether C-225 would be helpful, Joan agreed to my calling Harlan Waksal's office. Harlan came through again. We could start the treatment early next week.

The wait for C-225 was frustrating, but the week was fairly pleasant. Joan was relatively comfortable, in pretty good spirits, and enjoying time with Aaron, Johanna, Cathy, and close friends. The nurses and aides thought she was pretty special. Here was a woman who in all probability was dying, yet she remained engaged in the life of her family and friends, in good humor, and even willing to engage staff in serious conversation. Still a teacher, Joan was always willing to allow medical and nursing students to be present during procedures and even during discussions about sensitive matters. I recall the gratitude of one nursing student who was invited to stay in the room when Joan's oncologist reviewed the relative merits of implementing a "do not resuscitate" order. While heroics were not desired, we decided that day against doing so—mainly because we had not fully given up on the idea that Joan might have more time and because of my belief that a DNR communicates to some medical personnel that a less urgent level of care is needed. Ten days later we would add the DNR.

Knowing that Johanna would be visiting Joan, one of the night nurses brought two bunnies to Joan's room. While this was against hospital policy, no one seemed to mind that she was sneaking new life onto a cancer floor. It was great fun. We all enjoyed holding them and letting them hop around on the bed. (Cleanup was not as much fun.)

During this week, Joan videotaped messages to our kids, Cathy, and me. Joan was frustrated because she had found it so difficult to write letters to the kids. Johanna had expressed that she would like some letters in case Joan would not be present at major life events. I suggested considering videotaping what she wanted to say. Joan's face lit up.

We asked Jonathan Ball, a friend and skilled social worker, if he would conduct the interview. He was pleased to do this. A few days later he videotaped Joan's twenty-five-minute message to our children. I asked Jonathan how it went. "Almost nothing to it. I just started the camera, and Joan did everything else. I didn't have to ask a question. It was extraordinary." I thought Jonathan was being modest and also perhaps overstating Joan's performance. Not so. Two evenings later, after Jonathan had completed taping Joan's messages to Cathy and me, Joan asked if I would watch the tape and give her feedback about whether it was okay. I was amazed at how clearly Joan articulated her love for each of us, and her thoughts and concerns. I remain awed by how focused and centered her messages are and by her capacity to convey her love, her appreciation, and her guidance. These messages are each an ongoing source of strength and a reminder of what an amazing woman I was fortunate to marry.

Part of what she said to me, Cathy, and the kids follows.

[Eric] You'll feel me. I know you are going to feel me in the Adirondacks. And I know I am not leaving you. We have talked about that many, many times. And your spirituality gives me strength because I know that you know—on a really important and on a real, honest level—that I am not leaving you at all, not one little bit in terms of my spirit. That I am much more than this. That I know that you believe that on a plane that even our kids can't get to and maybe shouldn't be able to get to yet. I am sorry that I can't, I can't make that journey together, or whatever. . . . I just don't think that anybody has quite that privilege to do it together. And I am sorry that there are going to be really grief-stricken, lonely times. But I don't think I am going to be feeling them, so I think you can take great—I hope, I really hope you can take satisfaction—I know you have said many times you want me "in the flesh," and, of course, in some respects I'd rather be in the flesh. But I am also so ready to be released. And I really hope you can get to the joy of that feeling of being released for me. I know you respect me, and that feels wonderful. And you have all of my respect. And, umm, I just want you to know how much I love you.

And I don't know if I'll miss you or not because I don't know exactly where I'll be. I feel like I am going to be in many ways having the easier job. And I am going to be there. I am there, and if anybody in the world that I know will be listening, it's going to be you. I know you are going to have your ears wide open. You're so receptive and you're so intuitive and you're so spiritual . . . that even though I grieve for the grief you feel, I'll feel like it's cleansing. And I want you to feel my release as much as you can, even though it will be hard for you. . . . And I love you, you know that. I don't think I need to tell you I love you, but I will tell you anyway.

To Cathy she said,

It's just critical to me that you know from the bottom of my heart that you are the most precious, one of the most precious people in my life to me. That we will go on, that I know we will go on because I know . . . you have a deep spiritual sense of connection. And you'll be listening and I'll be there. And I think in many respects, more than anyone, you will have an appreciation of my release and a deep sense of relief for me. Because I know how wonderfully hard you have worked to protect me from those things that I don't want—like sometimes more pain or intervention or more western medicine, we call it. And I know that it has been very hard for Eric, being Eric, to accept me out of the flesh. And you have walked that very tight and balanced and difficult line in both supporting and understanding him—and really working to understand him and supporting and understanding my needs. . . . Anyway, I love you dearly. I'm there. And I think you know I'm there. And in our walks together, which will continue, I will be there and I know you will be open. I love you. You are just very precious. Thank you, Cathy.

And to the kids she ended her message:

I just adore you both. You taught me a lot. And I don't go in as much sadness as I go with a real feeling that, you know, that same feeling that I keep telling you. I am going to be there building those campfires for every one of you. Yours are going to be kind of last because you're coming last. But, anyway, I will be here and you know that. I am with you in every way but this bag of bones and blood and whatever—and that doesn't mean that much to me anymore—it's really, my spirit will be where you are. And I believe so much in you kids and am so proud of you, so very proud of you.

And go for walks, go for lots of walks and see me. I'll be there. No doubt I will be on your walks. That's going to be your closest place to get me. Be open to listening for me. Okay? Be open to my presence. Because I could be that deer swimming across the lake and if you are not open, you might miss me. But I think you will be open. Love you both.

Nearing Release

Well, as mentioned, we had again received permission to use C-225. But now there was a new more worrisome reason why it could not be used—Joan's liver enzymes had gone up, foreclosing the use of C-225. Neither Dr. Scalzo nor Imclone would authorize the use of the drug because her liver was close to failing.

Was this it? Was it now time to prepare for as comfortable a death as

ible? Joan was close to accepting death. I knew the likely outcome still had the belief, the hope, that we might get lucky. Dr. Scalzo, I think, believed continued treatment imprudent.

Joan agreed to talk with Dr. Kemeny. Dr. Kemeny said that she had seen some situations turn around, even at this advanced stage. One option might be to reactivate Joan's liver pump. By infusing the liver with FUDR, the enzymes might drop. If so, it would make sense to try C-225. The pump activation would be neither invasive nor uncomfortable for Joan. The upside was that she might get more time. The downside was that if FUDR did not work to improve the liver functions, then it would probably hasten liver failure and Joan's death. But as Dr. Kemeny explained, death by liver failure was not a very painful way to die. Joan decided this was a "win-win" situation! She decided to activate the pump.

Days passed pleasantly enough: our kids, Cathy, more friends, letters, my complaints about some of the student papers I was reading, and watching for signs of improved liver function.

One afternoon Aaron introduced Joan to his new girlfriend. Later that night, Joan cried as she told me how touched she was by Aaron wanting to introduce this lovely young woman to his mother.

April 29 was our twenty-second anniversary. I teared up as I looked through an arts and crafts shop in Armory Square for a gift. I found it hard to accept, but I knew this would be the last anniversary gift I bought for Joan—a deep turquoise ceramic tile with a shooting star embossed in its center. Later I wrote a note, and we celebrated our lives together. I cried; we probably cried together.

A couple of days had passed and the liver numbers were indeterminate. Maybe the decline had leveled off, we hoped. Another couple of days and the numbers looked a little better. Maybe we had turned a corner, we hoped.

May 4 was Johanna's sweet sixteenth birthday. It was very important to Joan that Johanna have a good recognition of her coming into womanhood. Cathy was especially attentive to Johanna. I returned to the same arts and crafts store and purchased a string of freshwater pearls, this time tearing because this would be the last birthday gift to come directly from Joan and me. We held a party in Joan's room, but there was a necessary undertone of sadness to this celebration.

On May 5, I wrote to friends:

> Several months ago, Joan said that if she must die, she hopes to teach those close to her that death does not have to be feared. We are learning this from her, though I can think of hundreds of other things I would rather learn from her. There is a small possibility that she will be able to start the chemo I mentioned in the previous email (C-225) and that it will prove beneficial. But no matter what, she is okay and in the hands of God.

The next test results showed further deterioration of Joan's liver. C-225 would not be used.

Release

I recall the remaining days as peaceful and immensely sad. Often with Cathy, Linda, and Michele, Joan would sit quietly, engaging in close conversation, punctuated by laughter and tears. Linda, a registered nurse, took over some of the care. Her exceptional wit was a welcomed distraction.

Around this time there were many other good-byes, in person and by telephone—George; my brother Steve, sister-in-law Sophie, and our nephew Matthew; Scott and Susan who came from Boston; Joan's cousins Bob and Ann Louise; Dennis and JoEllen; the Lux family; Johanna's friend Samantha; Alejandro, Brigit, Jonathan and Faith, and others.

On May 7 Joan talked with Dr. Scalzo about hastening her death by stopping all hydration and nutrition. She was at peace knowing that she would be allowed to drift into a coma and be kept relatively pain free as she moved toward death. Dr. Richard Cheney stopped by at some point, the doctor who had done his best to get Joan on C-225. Joan had previously complimented his choice of a tie, showing a dolphin jumping out of the ocean. He leaned over and presented the tie to her as a gift.

Joan put a call in to Nancy Kemeny. We long since learned that Dr. Kemeny, who first struck us as cold, was deeply caring of her patients. And the three of us had developed a close cooperative relationship. Joan expressed her appreciation to Dr. Kemeny. Both cried.

The hardest good-byes were with Aaron and Johanna. I do not know what words passed as each sat for final discussions with Joan, but I know Joan felt gratified by the love and closeness she felt with each. She was concerned with how the children would handle the loss but optimistic about the children she had raised and their capacity to live good, happy, and kind lives:

[Johanna,] I just think that what you said to Aunt Cathy the other night meant so much to me. That, you know, you're less concerned about my dying than on how I am feeling about my dying. That you're much less concerned about my dying, than being peaceful.

Joey, [you have] a lot of wisdom by [yourself] that [you are] beginning show. That it is how we feel about things and not what's happening; and how we manage things. And that's all along what I said I wanted you to learn. . . .

[Aaron,] that was a very, very important morning for me a couple of mornings ago, when we had time to really, really acknowledge our closeness in what I felt was just a very, very profound and honest way. [We acknowledged that] there's going to be grieving and that we are so connected. And I am your mother and you respect me and I respect so much that you respect me. . . .

And I hope you can continue to cry . . . I see that what our culture has done to men in many respects, I don't like. I don't like for you; I don't like for anyone else who is a sensitive man. And I feel like we don't allow men as we should to develop the kind of . . . sensitivity and courage that they need to develop in this culture. . . . It takes a lot more strength to show your feelings and to let yourself grieve, to get to the other side, which is real strength, I believe. And men seem to have less support for that. And I feel that we felt the other day that you were really feeling supported to do that. And you felt very comfortable the other day showing your mother every bit of grief and love that you have for me. I felt so complimented by it, and I felt so honored by it. . . .

I recall how in October 1998, as we drove to Sloan, Joan burst out crying as we listened to music from *Les Misérables*, the song in which Cosette's dying mother entrusts her upbringing to Jean Valjean. Joan, who had lost her mother when she was six, could not fathom leaving Johanna or Aaron without a mother. Now the time had come to take leave.

Earlier in this thirty-two-month marathon, Gussie Sorenson, the social worker at Hematology-Oncology, commented that "as you go along this journey, you may find that you redefine what you mean by 'hope.' " Yes, Gussie was right. Where once we had hoped for a reprieve, then a cure, and then some quality time, now Joan hoped for gentle release. And I turned my hope to there being more to life and love than what is visibly present.

Mary Jo, Cathy, Linda, and Michele were all present during the last few days and, of course, Aaron and Johanna. As Joan drifted in and out of consciousness, she spoke of feeling her mother's presence, of feeling she was going home. We began making preparations for the funeral, identifying a cemetery, and asking Terry Culbertson if she would officiate.

The hospital staff were exceptionally kind and concerned. A pain-free death was now the goal, the hope. During the final nights, I often stood by her bed and held her hand, telling her how much I loved her and coaching, "It's okay, Hon, it's time to let go. It's time to die."

On May 10, Mary Jo and Linda stayed overnight in the room with Joan and me. At the slightest sign of discomfort, we would request more morphine for Joan. The next day, Joan's last, was peaceful. That night I slept sitting up in a chair next to her, my left hand on her chest, my head by her side and my right hand on her head. I would wake and ask Reeja Luthra, the night nurse we had gotten to know, to give Joan more medication to make her more comfortable. She did. In the morning I woke to Reeja standing over Joan, still warm. "Is she gone?" I asked. Reeja checked Joan's heartbeat. Joan had been released. She was at peace and the room felt peaceful. But how missed she was and still is.

AUTUMN ROSE ELEGY

You've gone to the secret world.
Which way is it? You broke the cage

and flew. You heard the drum that
calls you home. You left this hu-

miliating shelf, this disorienting
desert where we're given wrong

directions. What use now a crown?
You've become the sun. No need for

a belt: you've slipped out of your
waist! I have heard that near the

end you were eyes looking at soul.
No looking now. You live inside

the soul. You're the strange autumn
rose that led the winter wind in

by withering. You're rain soaking
everywhere from cloud to ground. No

bother of talking. Flowing silence
and sweet sleep beside the Friend.

—Jalal ad-Din Rumi (thirteenth-century Sufi sage)

7

Epilogue

LIVING AFTER DEATH

✍ Four years later and I deeply miss Joan, my life's anticipated partner. Four years later and I look forward to life.

MEMORIAL SERVICE

The memorial service was in our backyard on May 16, 2001.

Three hundred people crowded under a large tent to share Joan's
life and death. Family and friends from past homes—Waltham, Natick
and Baltimore, Buffalo and New York City—Syracuse friends, neighbors, colleagues, and some health care providers, students and teachers
from our children's high schools, professional friends from Wheelock,
Boston College, Maryland, and elsewhere.

A simple unadorned pine casket, podium at its side, paralleled the
front of our deck, holding what Joan called "this bag of flesh and
bones"—the body of the woman we loved so much. A solo violinist
played in the background.

"Turn, Turn, Turn"—a prayer, a song—that reminds of life's cycles,
was special to Joan. Our Natick neighbor, Mary Ellen Whitaker, sang it
at the start of Johanna's bat mitzvah. I asked Mary Ellen if she might
sing this to open our service. Unable to take the day off from work, she
felt terrible. She called back with an idea. It worked. Mary Ellen and an

instrumental accompanist cut a special CD in honor of Joan—an extraordinary rendition I have since listened to hundreds of times.

Mary Ellen's voice commenced the service. After the song, Reverend Culbertson stepped forth in the silence:

> Good afternoon everyone. I'm Reverend Terry Culbertson and I was asked by Joan Kingson to officiate at her service. It says in the book of Ecclesiastes, "To everything there is a season and a time for every purpose under heaven." And they speak about the harmonious balance of nature and life, how things weigh themselves out against each other, from life until death, laughing and time to weep and plant and reaping. And this afternoon we come together to give honor and to celebrate the life of a very special woman, Joan Fernbach Kingson—a person who lived life and stretched her time to the fullest. . . .
>
> We gather together to give thanks for her life, for her time on this earth, to acknowledge her death and the fact that she is sorely missed. And then as her community, to recall what gives us hope and faith in this life and in the life to come.
>
> Whether you are family or friends, or just happen to know Joan through the children, it seems that anybody who met Joan knew she was a special person. And, whatever your relationship, I hope you will be able to join in with us in both laughter and tears to share because, you see, Joan planned this service, she loved nature, she loved the outdoors, she loved her backyard, and she wanted each one of you to be comfortable at home with her today. She picked out the music and . . . before we close, she has a few words to tell us.

Like Joan, the service had structure and character, and it was informal. It did justice to Joan's spirit, her life's commitments and the special gift Joan had of being very present—as mother, wife, sister, and friend. Family and friends set forth recollections of Joan. With humor and love, Mary Jo told of how growing up as Joan's younger sister was not always easy. Yes, Joan had a mischievous side. She had an extraordinary loving and generous side that Aaron spoke of in his eulogy. As Johanna would later tell the student body and teachers of her high school, Joan "accomplished so much in her last years because she chose to spend them living rather than dying despite her failing body." And, on this day, too, she remained a caring teacher—delivering, through the spirit of the event, the message that death doesn't need to be feared, especially if you have lived a good and caring life.

Johanna's track coach, Bill Aris, reflected on Joan's grace and commitment to her children, recalling how even in the winter prior to her death she managed to go to Johanna's indoor track meets. Natick neighbors talked of Joan's strength, humor, and love of walking. My sister-in-law, Sophie Glasgow Kingson, recalled her warmth and interest in Matthew. Johanna's friends spoke of how valued, how heard they always felt they were by Joan. As the service ended, twelve women carried Joan's casket to the vehicle that would take her to Oakwood Cemetery. Unusual, but nice to have women do this, some commented. Only natural and certainly something Joan would have liked.

The violinist, a Syracuse Symphony musician, joined us at the cemetery, playing as 120 or so people assembled (the others who attended the service had taken a wrong turn and never made it to the cemetery). I appreciated that he had made himself available on such short notice and was delighted to have a violin present at the service and now the grave. He had done a wonderful job, though one selection was not your normal graveside fare. As we waited, I heard the melody of "Hava Nagilah"—a festive Israeli song. I recall smiling to myself and thinking that Joan would find this departure from protocol very amusing.

Terry led us in prayer, sharing with my brother, Steve, the lead in saying the Mourner's Kaddish. During the memorial service, Terry had read and likened Joan to the "Lupine Lady," who brought beauty into the world by spreading seeds. Now she would close the service by casting lupine seeds on Joan's grave, from which new beauty might grow. We returned the earth to Joan's grave and left.

REFLECTIONS

Aaron's Eulogy

Mom, I'm proud of you. I'm proud of your strength and courage in living, and, at too young of an age, your strength and courage in dying. I'm proud of how you so generously and quietly gave yourself to everyone in your life, never asking or expecting anything in return. But most importantly, I am proud to be your son.

As you have said to me over and over, we share a special relationship. One filled with love and concern for one another, and strengthened by mutual respect and an unwavering trust. A relationship complete with a bond too strong to ever break.

Speaking of special relationships, you brought out the best in my father, and he brought out the best in you. I can only hope and pray that, one day, I will experience the kind of marriage and love that you two share. A marriage filled with hope, trust, and understanding. A love that grew with every new experience, hurdle, and hard time; a love so boundless that it changed both of you into better, more whole people.

Both by yourself and with my father, you have given and taught me so much. In mourning your death, I find myself in a state of both grief and happiness. Grief because it is only healthy and natural for a son to grieve when his mother dies. Happiness because the only memories that I have of my childhood are beautiful, uplifting, and loving ones. For this reason, as well as an infinite number of others, you will always be with me. I promise to forever hold the strength and love that you have given me close to my heart and share it with others in your giving spirit. As a token of this, I am dedicating all of my future work and affiliations with the Boys and Girls Clubs to you, Mom. As you know, the clubs are a part of who I am and who I strive to be, just as you are. I hope to continue to make you proud.

While I will always strive to be like you in one way, I know that I am already you in a different sense. I am you when I reach out to someone in need of a loving hand, I am you when I sit back and intuitively hear a friend out for as long as they want for me to listen. I am you when I need my time to be alone, to think about things greater than myself. I am you when I am at my best, thinking of everyone except for myself.

So please, surround me occasionally on walks or in the Adirondacks, guide me with yet another silent conversation or unspoken understanding. And please know, too, that while I can't explain how much I'll miss you, we will always be together. You are too much a part of me by now for it to be any other way.

With everlasting love and gratitude,

Bear, your son forever.

Mary Jo's Eulogy

It was not always easy being Joan's little sister.

Growing up, Joan would pretend to be the bogeyman. Late at night, she would sneak into the room and scare the daylights out of me. I always felt that Joan did things better than I did. She was more athletic, she studied harder, she got better grades, and she was more popular. Joan was always the president, be it the student council or whichever club interested her. Joan lived life with intensity.

I shared a room with Joan for the first fifteen years of my life. Joan would not only clean and organize her half of the room, but she would organize and clean my half of the room. As a result I hold Joan partially responsible for my disorganization as an adult today.

Through the years I learned some very important lessons from Joan. She taught me the art of nun handling. This was of utmost importance when attending a Catholic girls school. Joan taught me never to go to a supermarket without buying Vienna fingers.

Joan taught me to appreciate a good novel. Joan would circulate the most interesting books. Family and friends were always excited to receive one of Joan's latest selections. Joan taught me an appreciation of nature and the benefits of a good long walk. Joan taught me to see the beauty in the hearts of others.

Joan taught me not to be afraid of living a full life. And later, Joan taught me to not even fear death.

Some years back, my son was critically ill. Joan was always there helping out. That was Joan, offering her help and love to others as they navigated troubled waters.

Over the last three years, Joan navigated her own troubled waters. She did so with dignity and grace, opening her heart, allowing others to come to peace with her passing. As I watched her during the last several weeks, Joan grew more beautiful and peaceful as she neared land's end.

I would like to share this excerpt of a poem by Mary Oliver called "In Blackwater Woods." I mailed this to Joan about a year ago and she told me how much it meant to her:

. . . .
Every year
everything
I have ever learned

in my lifetime
leads back to this: the fires
and the black river of loss
whose other side

is salvation,
whose meaning
none of us will ever know.
To live in this world

you must be able
to do three things:
to love what is mortal;
to hold it

against your bones knowing
your own life depends on it;
and, when the time comes to let it go,
to let it go.
   —Mary Oliver

Joan told me two weeks ago that she loved me and that she would always be my big sister. I would not have it any other way.

Johanna Reflects on Walks at Wellesley Pond with Her Mom
(February 6, 2002)

"Your choice! High or low?" I heard this set of choices often, yet it made me feel important each time my mom asked me to choose the path of travel. It was in my realm of power to decide whether we took the high or low path for the first 70 meters of our walk. Ultimately, we ended up at the same spot, but it was up to me to dictate how we got there. When the high and low path diverged, we continued on our two-and-a-half-mile route around Wellesley College. Over the course of twelve years (the duration of time in which I lived in Boston), I must have gotten over five hundred miles worth of exercise from that same two and a half miles!

Splash! "Joey, careful!" Another one of my mom's favorite lines. She was obligated by her motherhood to say this, even though it was obviously a hopeless cause. The clanking of my heavy, saturated boots echoed throughout the woods as I ran across the coiled metal drain pipe. "There it is! Look Mom! It came through!" At that moment I was met with a warm, sincere smile. It is not her smile that I remember her for, rather, that deep twinkle in her eye that functioned as a window into her soul.

On the days of our long walks, I was the one who put the twinkle in her eye. She was full of joy, admiration, and excitement with the idea of having me, her daughter. At the time, I believed she was truly amazed at my trick of putting a log on one side of the drain pipe and miraculously watching it come out the other side. Looking back, I realize that the log was not what my mother was watching at all, though my sole focus was not to miss its entrance out of the other side of the tunnel. Her eyes took in the wonderful scene of her daughter at play, for she truly loved and appreciated her role as a mother, caretaker, and provider. The twinkle was not a reflection of light, instead a passage for this light into her body, mind, and soul.

Years earlier, when my mom was a little girl, she unknowingly put this same twinkle into her father's eyes. For a moment between the time when the sun left the daytime sky and the moon illuminated the night sky, time froze for my mom and her father. Buffalo's city blocks seemed to go on forever, though it was never long enough for those two. Each step they trod functioned as an escape for her father from hardships, like a mini vacation or getaway. It is known that all vacations must come to an end, and at the end of their walk he was thrown back into his destructive cycle of alcohol abuse.

Those simultaneous steps along the crooked, cracked, weathered city blocks that my mom's father took with his daughter at his side formed a bond that tied those two together into eternity. A bond that was passed on to future generations. I often wonder if they both would not have been better off if they had been on a never-ending walk; one in which they enjoyed each other's company and walked right past the hardships of life, for they both suffered so many. Instead, they used walks as

I now do. Walks are a break from the hardships and a celebration of all the wonderful instances that life is made up of.

"Mom, how do you think they get to the way top of the tree to shape it?" We were greeted by these monstrosities of trees that took on the most unnatural shapes of triangles and domes. Not a branch was out of place, for it was clear that whoever the sculptor, he made sure to trim and re-trim often. In my head I envisioned a small man climbing up the branches, trimming and tweaking as he went along. I know now that there was some sort of stepladder involved for the other option is really quite absurd. On an earlier walk, I had described to my mom, with no lack of enthusiasm or detail, how I believed this tree shaping was accomplished. Yet it still remained a mystery to me how the little man got to the tip top of the tree, for the branches are much smaller at the top. I feared he might fall, even though I didn't picture him to weigh much over ninety pounds.

My mom saw the spark, excitement, and energy that I received from hypothesizing about sculpting trees. Rather than inform me on the wonders of modern technology, she allowed my imagination to run wild. It would have been easiest and incredibly convenient for her to shut down my wild and creative side, which, at times, bordered on overbearing and imperious. Though many people would have preferred for her to act in such a manner, this was something she refused to do. My creativity and imagination is the greatest gift that she ever gave me, and, believe me, it took an incredible amount of energy and patience on her part. She was able to help me find ways to channel my energy. My mom succeeded in her goals, for I use the gift of walking to release energy, creativity, and emotions. "Joey, I have never seen how they get to the way top of the tree to shape it. Your guess is as good as mine." What a perfect response to my question!

"Are we almost there?" I probably could have drawn a map of the exact spot on the lake which we were at. We had approximately one-fifth of the walk remaining, and I knew it and my mom knew that I knew it. I only asked because it seemed natural that I would do so, for my legs had started aching and I was looking to my mom for comfort, empathy, and encouragement. I began to envision the ride home. The comforting and familiar sounds of my mom switching gears in our Volvo as it huffed and puffed up our hill. My daydreaming was broken by a comforting voice reassuring me, "Yes, Joey. We are almost there."

It is funny how at the time I only focused on completing that last portion of our walk as quickly as possible, though right now, as I walk beside my good friend Sam, I want more than words can express to be completing that last one-fifth of my walk with my mom by my side. To be lost in a walk with her, our walk, sounds like the sweetest of dreams to me. I find that she truly has become a part of me, for my speech and actions mimic hers so closely. My mom's presence is so vivid on the walks I take today. Though she may not physically be walking next to me, I know she surrounds me on these walks. I breathe in the air she is a part of, and, at this time, I lose myself in the walk of my ancestors. I give Sam the option of which direction we shall walk around the lake. A twinkle enters my eye as I say, "Your choice! Right or left?"

FOUR YEARS LATER

Fifty-two months have passed since we covered Joan's grave. They have been difficult months. Joan said she thought I would probably have the harder task once she was gone. I do not know whether this is true, but I hope it is, as much of the time since her death has been very difficult. And yet, I am pleased to be alive, and I am optimistic that my path— which will always be connected with Joan's—is leading me to a rich and full life.

Many times in the past four years I have wished I were with Joan. I have and will continue to search out ways to communicate with her. I carry a belief—but one that I am far from certain is true—that in some way our souls, our energies are connected, and that we will be in more direct communication again. In part, this is a result of the Reiki experience; in part, a feeling, a hope.

I had hoped to make direct contact with Joan, but I have not had an experience that assures me she is there, waiting. The closest I got was a waking dream, what some might call a vision, when Johanna and I first visited our Adirondack home shortly after Joan died. There she was, in a red jacket and old jeans, clapping her hands and saying, "Come on, up and at 'em; there's work to do"—as if she was about to enlist me in some project in the yard. Then there was a dream, a very realistic dream, where I was diagnosed with advanced cancer. "That's okay," I said, "Then I will get to see Joan."

I value my grief. It keeps me connected to Joan. How sad it would be to commit to a lifetime with someone and not feel a deep, painful loss when they are gone.

I have spent many hours at her grave. I didn't have a plan for it, but it has turned into a beautiful setting. Shortly after she died, friends from Natick, Joe Citrone and his son Mark, paid us a visit. They wanted to visit the grave. Still relatively bare, I had planted two lilies at her feet, "Joan Flowers," which I will tell you about shortly. Joe commented that we ought put some boulders near the flowers or they might be mowed over. The three of us collected some large rocks. I liked the way they looked.

Since then, I have ringed her grave with rocks—large and small. Rocks from Chapel Pond and the Cascade Lakes outside Keene, New York, where we often swam. Rocks from Adirondack streams, from Puerto Rico, Costa Rica, and Mexico. A large natural granite boulder—inscribed "Fernbach Kingson"—marks the plot. And below her headstone, white pebbles spell out "Joan." Cathy and I have planted bulbs and biennials, and I take pleasure in caring for the grave. I often think of Joan's bemusement that her death finally got me started on gardening.

At Green Lakes and Mill Run Parks, we have placed simple wooden benches. My favorite sits in a small grove, a pine-scented chapel close to the lake, with words from *Les Misérables* inscribed—"To love another person is to see the face of God." I have sat quietly there and walked the Green Lakes trying to feel her presence. I hear her say, "I am here, Eric: I am always here." But I do not know who is speaking—my hopes and dreams? Or ours?

Kind words and notes, donations in her memory to the Boys and Girls Clubs of Syracuse, a blood drive organized by my Syracuse colleagues—we experienced many welcomed expressions of sympathy. One childhood friend, John Jiler, wrote:

> I guess you are feeling a million things right now. I hope one of them is all the love that was under that tent. It was one of the most powerful things I've ever experienced. I felt so privileged to be included. . . .
>
> I am so curious about what will happen next for you, Eric. A strange new time is beginning with many dark patches but probably with many unexpected bright ones too. You are sailing on waters that very few of us know, or will know. Maybe that's where Joan's campfires will come into play; to comfort you, but to keep you off the shoals. I know she doesn't want you lighting yours for a long time.
>
> Clearly she spent a lot of energy to see that the three of you would be all right. The surprise was that she did it for the three hundred of us too! Everyone I spoke to afterward was exhilarated and emboldened by it. Nobody was depressed. It was a wondrous gift.

Beautiful yellow lilies—termed "The Joan Flowers" by our Natick friends who planted them in her memory—bloom in late summer throughout our Natick neighborhood and elsewhere where our friends are found, a visible reminder of her strength and spirit of friendship. And Joan's spirit of caring friendship lives well through occasional "girls' weekends." Planned by Joan as she died, Cathy, Linda, Mary Jo, and Michele take these weekends as welcomed opportunities to shower

Johanna with stories, laughter, and love. And through fond memories and lessons gently taught.

Just as this is not the book I ever expected to write, neither is the path I have taken since Joan's death what I could possibly have anticipated.

Among Joan's many gifts was her assurance that if I fell in love after she died, that she would be pleased—"It would be an expression of our love, Eric." She understood, better than I, that finding love after the death of a beloved spouse is a gift, not competitive with prior love that still lives but having much in common with the complexity and joy parents feel for a child born second—deep and true and bewildering in its capacity to engage so much of you so quickly. Many times I have thought of the kindness and generosity of her love.

Not surprisingly, these past four years have been difficult for Aaron and Johanna, nineteen and sixteen when Joan died, and far too young to be introduced to such grief. Kind people, strong-willed and sensitive, the piercing pain of their loss will soften, though many warm memories of Joan will always serve as reminder and ache for memories missed.

There is much to tell of their experiences, but I leave that for them to share in their own way. Trusting in a good future for both, their presence enriches my life and I look forward to sharing what is around the corner for them.

Love and kindness—God's grace entwined in our humanity—make life worth living. Trusting in a good tomorrow, I am excited to engage my future while keeping the love and richness of life with Joan, and the family we raised, always by my side and in my soul. And when I see those campfires burning on a future shore, I will approach their warmth with gratitude, an open heart, and much curiosity.

APPENDIXES

FINAL NOTE OF APPRECIATION

Practical Lessons for Negotiating Cancer

𝕵𝕽 The main body of this book is a narrative of Joan's experience and mine, as her life partner, as we negotiated thirty-two months of cancer. I switch gears in this appendix and in appendix B. Although *Lessons from Joan* is not a "how to" book, I am aware that some reading this book are, as Joan and I were, engaged in responding to their own or a loved one's life-threatening illness. Drawing on Joan's and my experiences, these appendices present lessons and selected tools for negotiating cancer or other life-threatening illnesses.

Appendix A briefly summarizes lessons for negotiating the health care system and for living well with cancer or other life-threatening illnesses. Two essays—one authored by Joan's sister Catherine Fernbach and myself, and the other by my daughter, Johanna—are included because they illustrate these lessons.

LESSONS FOR NEGOTIATING THE HEALTH CARE SYSTEM

Experience is often the best teacher, even if you are not seeking knowledge. Unfortunately, Joan and I were taught quite a bit during our thirty-two months of negotiating the health care system. Since each person's experience is unique, what may have worked for Joan or me is not necessarily right for others. Still, I summarize some practical lessons here, thinking they may be beneficial to some.

Understand that you are in a marathon, not a sprint. When a cancer diagnosis is made, the tendency is to want to do something about it. Right away! But as we learned, it was important to take time to understand treatment options, to select an oncologist, to seek second and third opinions, to collect our emotions, to put supports in place for our children and ourselves.

Take time to explore carefully treatment choices. Get second and third opinions. Especially during initial diagnosis, it's important to take a deep breath and not rush into treatment without being sure that necessary diagnostic information is complete. Try to keep as many options open as possible. Understand that outstanding physicians may not always have the knowledge that highly specialized docs at regional cancer centers have. As was the case for us, a surgeon like Dr. Fong, who may perform 150 liver surgeries annually, may be able to do liver surgeries that excellent general surgeons would not consider possible. Understanding this, knowledgeable and secure physicians welcome the insights and suggestions of other reputable specialists. If your treating doctor is not open to second or third opinions, then you may want to find another doctor.

Information is your friend, especially good information presented in ways you can hear. It is difficult to hear that you have cancer, or that you are no longer in remission, or that there is a "suspicious" finding. Waiting for test results is difficult as they may confirm suspicions of a major health problem. For many of us, these are periods of great anxiety and fear. In the face of such information, ignorance may seem like bliss. But lack of information robs you of opportunities to effectively treat a disease, limits choices about how to use your time, takes away opportunities to share some of life's most intimate moments with those you love.

There are many ways of gathering information—from health care providers, from others who have walked down similar paths, from the Internet (see appendix B) and research journals. Assess what information you need to make good choices. Assess how you would like that information given to you. Do you want to receive test results as soon as possible (for example, a "wet" read from a radiologist right after a CT scan)? Do you want to know the survival data or not? Think about whether you might benefit from gathering information available on the Internet. Talk with your health care providers. Be clear about your needs. Be clear that while information is your friend, it may not always be correct.

You are not a statistic. The data that yield estimates of survival time, progression-free survival, or reoccurrence are based on past research. The data refer to averages. You are not an average; you are a person. No one can predict how long you will live or what the outcomes of an intervention will be. You may (or you may not) find knowledge of survival data useful to your decision making. But, no matter what, do not treat yourself or allow yourself to be treated as a number.

Learn to ride the "roller coaster." In the world of cancer, at least the part of that world that we inhabited, we learned that things are often not as bad as they at first seem. Conversely, often they are not as good as they might appear. Expect many ups and downs.

Bite your tongue, cool your heels, keep your eye on the target. Before Joan's illness, I was much quicker to anger when kept waiting for long periods of time for an appointment or when faced with inconsiderate treatment. Now that the stakes were high, however, I learned to pick and choose my battles carefully. I also recognized that physician schedules are not easily maintained. The extra time an oncologist gives to a patient at a crucial time or that a surgeon spends to complete surgery may throw off their schedules. Sometimes you or a family member are that patient that needed the extra time.

In most situations, it is not going to help you (or the person you love) to be defined as a problem. There are, of course, times when you need to be assertive or take a strong position. Rule of thumb: think it through and, to the extent possible, be measured in your response.

Consider participating in clinical trials. Before making treatment decisions, be sure to explore whether you might benefit from a clinical trial. Learn about available trials, the promise of the interventions being studied, and relative risks. Remember, just as there may be risks associated with participation in a trial, there may also be risks associated with bypassing the opportunity to participate.

Don't assume that health care providers "don't care." Or that biomedical researchers are not concerned about their patients and others suffering from disease. It's easy to stereotype health care providers, especially researchers, as cold and unfeeling. No doubt some are. But mostly they are human, like you and me. Some are emotionally distant, often a means to defend against the pain that comes when a patient does not do as well as they hoped. Some nurses may appear rushed, even brisk, not having enough time to fully engage the physical and emotional needs of patients. Unfortunately, they often are rushed not because of a lack of concern but due to the extraordinary pressures on nurses in today's managed care environment. Truth is, most would rather have more time for patient care. As for people involved in research, while they are committed to caring for individual patients in their studies, the source of their commitment often comes from deep desire to find ways to ameliorate, cure, or prevent harmful diseases.

The trade-off between treatment and quality of life may not always be what you anticipate. Avoid dichotomous thinking about the implications of treatment. Aggressive interventions do not necessarily compromise quality of life. Doing nothing may actually compromise quality. Or there may be compromises, and, assessed against the alternatives, you may deem them acceptable.

Keep good records and communicate. Maintain a running record of your illness history, from diagnoses through treatments. Encourage health care providers to be in contact with each other and to share information. (See appendix B for examples of tools we used.)

Bring an extra set of ears to critical meetings with health care providers. Under the best of circumstances, it is difficult to absorb medical information, and it's even harder when the information you are taking in raises your anxiety. If you are in the midst of diagnosis or critical treatment decisions, it is often beneficial to ask someone you trust to join you at critical meetings, to listen, to take notes, to be a little more dispassionate than you might be.

Be tenacious. Gather information. Contact people who may be of assistance to you or your loved one. Assume that you can access needed treatments. More often than not, where there is a will, there is a way. And as they say, "You can gather more bees with honey than with vinegar."

Consider using an advanced directive or health care proxy. Everyone bears the risk of being in a position in which they are unable to give verbal directions about the type of treatment they want or do not want. Whether young or old, healthy or ill, having a will in effect is always a good idea. Similarly, regardless of health status, it is a good idea to have an advanced directive about the type of care you would like and/or designating someone as your proxy in the event you are unable to give expression to your views. Also, you should be familiar with the implications of and your own feelings about the use of "Do Not Resuscitate" (DNR) orders.

Have someone stay with you at the hospital. Hospitals are busy places. They are also lonely places. No matter how good the care, it's often helpful to have someone to run errands, to keep track of scheduled medications, to keep you company, to advocate on your behalf if necessary.

Do not hesitate to say "thank you." It is important for health care providers to understand that patients and families value what is being done for them. Joan was very appreciative of care provided at Crouse and intended to write a note of appreciation, an intent that led her sister Catherine Fernbach and I to give expression to Joan's and our appreciation in a letter to the *Syracuse Post-Standard*:

"HEALTH CARE THAT WORKED TO THE END"

(Op-Ed Letter in the *Syracuse Post-Standard*)
Eric Kingson and Catherine Fernbach

Our family understands how important competent health care is for patients and their family members living with a life-threatening disease. And, as the 15-part newspaper series "Living with Dying in America" highlights, we also understand how needed and valued compassionate end-of-life care is, by those who die and family members who live on.

Joan Fernbach Kingson was diagnosed with metastatic

colon cancer in October 1998. She underwent several major surgeries and many chemotherapies in Syracuse, New York, at Memorial Sloan-Kettering Cancer Center in New York City and at the University of Massachusetts Medical Center in Worcester, Massachusetts. She did not receive the 5, 10 or 30 extra years that she sought, but she did receive the two most important years in her and our lives, time that was very well cherished and used. And six months past her death, while we remain very sad, we are immensely grateful for the type of care she received from the beginning to the end of her cancer.

You learn a lot when you spend as much time as we have in health care settings with someone you love.

We saw highly committed and extraordinarily busy medical researchers, oncologists, surgeons, nurse practitioners and others listen carefully to their patients and communicate with respect. You learn the importance of trusting dedicated oncologists such as Syracuse's Tony Scalzo and Sloan-Kettering's Nancy Kemeny. You learn that highly skilled surgeons can be very human in their interaction with patients and families; that aggressive experimental interventions can improve quality of life; that little kindnesses of secretaries, physicians, nurses and parking lot attendants matter.

We saw, firsthand, how hard nurses and nurses aides work. Seven or eight patients (sometimes 10 on weekends) assigned to a nurse or nurse's aide may not sound like much to the layperson or, sadly, to those financing our health care systems. But when you have patients with complex needs, the responsibility is—as Joan would say—"daunting."

We saw care that reflects deep respect for the dignity of patients and family. Like Joan, at some point during our lives, nearly all of us will be challenged to accept the help of family, friends and "strangers" with the most personal types of care. Joan did not feel diminished, and could accept—sometimes even enjoy—this care because it was given freely and with respect.

After a thirty-one day admission, Joan died in room 4005 at Syracuse's Crouse Hospital, comfortably and without fear, in the arms and hearts of family and friends. She received the finest care possible from "Four-South's" nurse-practitioner, nurses, nurses' aides, chaplains, social worker, maintenance staff, secretaries and volunteers. And, as was always the case during her 32-month illness, the oversight and care from physicians, nurses and other medical professionals was first rate, in every way.

Joan truly was not afraid of dying. Given the progression of the cancer, she saw death as a release from, as she put it, "this bag of bones" and as a welcomed transition to a different place.

A few days before dying, she asked that all treatment, including hydration and nutrition, be stopped and that things only be done to keep her pain free and comfortable. Rather than go home to die, she chose to stay in Crouse Hospital. She was and our family is thankful for a health care system that worked for her. And we greatly appreciate that Crouse Hospital allowed room 4005 to be her and our last home together.

We lost someone we deeply love. Days, weeks and now months have past. Reflecting on her illness and last month, we recognize that this loss was made immeasurably easier by the type of care Joan received, especially at the end of her life.

Eric Kingson lives in Syracuse, New York, and is Joan's husband. Catherine Fernbach lives in Somerville, Massachusetts, and is Joan's sister. Joan Fernbach Kingson, MED, BSN, was a child-life educator and taught about working with children and families in health care settings.

LESSONS FOR LIVING WELL WITH CANCER

Cancer and other life-threatening illnesses, uninvited teachers, leave those they visit with new understandings of what's important and at the core of the human experience. I'll discuss some of these lessons now, ending with a speech by our daughter, Johanna, where she passed on to students at her high school what she learned from how her mom handled her illness.

Self-help is good, but don't blame yourself. The self-help literature is replete with suggestions for preventing, warding off, curing, and learning to live with many illnesses. Joan and I read some of the books on dealing with cancer. They were often helpful. And I believe Joan's walking and positive approach to living in spite of the cancer added time to her life. Such activities certainly added quality.

However, some self-help approaches imply that not only can you cure your illness but that it is somehow "your fault" if you do not. Joan greatly resented and rejected this message. As she might say, "Look, you can live well, exercise, eat lots of broccoli, and have a good outlook and still die from cancer!" She was similarly clear when told that she "failed chemo." "No," she would say, "Chemo failed me."

You can control the little things, and they matter. Truth is, many of the big things in life are out of your control. You may not be able to prevent your company from closing or cancer from striking. But you can control your responses to such events. And, as my cousin Jim Kramon mentioned, there are many little things in life you can control: taking time with your loved ones, looking up to enjoy passing clouds on a warm summer day, or going to a baseball game, play, or concert . . .

Learn to accept care from those you love. It's a gift to you and to them. Learning to give, to care for others, is an important part of our development as human beings. As infants, we depend entirely on others. By adulthood, more often than not, we give more than we receive as parents, as members of our community. Some people, like Joan, excel at giving to others but have difficulty accepting the care of others. Over the course of her illness—and without loss of strength, dignity, or humanity—Joan learned to accept, even at times enjoy, the care of health care providers, family, and friends. Her comfort and grace in accepting care with appreciation was a gift that brought her closer to her caregivers.

Take care of yourself and your family. No surprise: being confronted with a life-threatening illness is extraordinarily stressful. Whether you are diagnosed with such an illness or giving care to someone who is, find ways to care for yourself and those you love. Embrace small pleasures, pace yourself, develop good relationships with health care providers, and "don't sweat the small stuff." Find humor wherever you can. You and those around you need it more than ever. Humor and laughter may not cure cancer, but they can give expression to and reinforce a healthy spirit. Accept and acknowledge the concern of family and friends. And consider seeking professional support for you and your family from chaplains, therapists, and other counselors.

Kindnesses—large and small—matter to you and matter to others. Simple kindness, like humor, gives expression to and reinforces the human spirit. The nurse who kissed Joan's forehead in advance of a feared procedure or the physician who gave Joan his tie as she neared death touched us in special ways. Joan's capacity to get outside her pain, to move beyond her anxiety, and to engage with interest the concerns of some of the nursing students, aides, and others giving care—even as she approached death—touched others deeply. Life-threatening illnesses challenge the understandings and rhythms of our lives. Kindness, given and received, provides the opportunity to transcend human suffering and find meaning in the capacity of the human spirit to endure.

Leave a videotape, letter, or other message for those you love. As someone who lost his father at age thirteen, I have often hoped, even as an adult, to find a note from him: some advice about life, some stories of importance to him . . . In contrast, I have deeply appreciated my mother's forethought in leaving a long letter for her sons. And Joan's eloquent video good-bye is part of her treasured legacy to our family. Consider leaving a message for those you love. By the way, you don't have to be ill or proximate to death to do this.

Do not underestimate the effects on kids of a parent's illness. As I look back on this time and think about how threatening and ultimately devastating the loss of a parent is, I wish we had better prepared Aaron and Johanna for the depth of the loss they would experience. We, especially Joan, tried. But we were also invested in maintaining some normality to their high school years, maybe too invested. And, while not keeping any information from them, we did not want to rob them or ourselves of the hope that we might have many years in front of us. No suggestions for others here, just the observation that no matter which route is chosen, the pain and sadness that children must bear when a parent dies runs very deep.

Recognize some special "opportunities" that are a by-product of cancer. No, I am not suggesting that cancer and other life-threatening illnesses are gifts: just that they provide opportunities and insights you would not normally have. There are potential advantages of having the blinders of everyday life—the fantasy that keeps awareness of our impermanence at bay—ripped away by a cancer diagnosis. Everyone born goes down life's path to death. Some arrive there sooner than others. Some live better because they recognize the limitations that life brings. Cancer can provide people with the opportunity to reflect on the meaning of their lives, to renew their commitments, to grow in ways never expected, to have time to repair relationships, to say full good-byes to those they love. Growth and learning and teaching do not stop with a cancer diagnosis, not even with death's approach. Joan learned much in her thirty-two months of cancer, especially about how loved and worthy of love she was. She taught much to our family and others—about dying, living, and courage, about the endurance of the human spirit.

Living in hope trumps fear. Fear is not an unreasonable response to a cancer diagnosis, especially advanced cancer. Mark Twain observed that he spent much of his life worrying about things that never happened. Similarly, living in too much fear—even when reality-based—can ruin the time you have, time that may stretch out to decades.

In the course of Joan's cancer, we learned to live in hope. Living in hope is not synonymous with blind denial, with sticking one's head in the sand. Hope, as Gussie Sorensen first suggested, evolved over the course of the illness, from hope for a cure, to hope for remission for extra time, to hope for a "good" death. Joan's appreciation of her walks, our children, her friends and books were expressions and outgrowths of the hope. My pleasure in her smile, her humor, and courage part of the hope.

And hope drove our faith in good lives for our children and the permanence of our union. There was still much fear, but we learned that living in hope gave us much life, more than we could ever have expected.

Johanna's Talk to Her High School

Johanna gave this speech in March 2002 before an assembly of students at her high school as part of a fundraiser for Camp Good Days and Special Times, a camp for kids and families that have experienced cancer.

My mother was diagnosed with colon cancer in September of '98. Given the severity of her diagnosis, it seemed unlikely that she would live beyond six months. My mother made the choice not to focus on what had happened to others with similar diagnoses but to instead approach this battle as an individual. It was this attitude that allowed her to live much longer than any physician could have predicted. I would often hear her say, "I am doing my darndest to buy whatever time I can as long as I can maintain a high quality of life." It was in her last years that she derived the most meaning from her life and was able to deeply touch the lives of so many.

My mother was able to accomplish so much in her last years because she chose to spend them living rather than dying despite her failing body. Her ability to teach, love, and provide for others, while simultaneously struggling with fears incomprehensible to most, is what made her truly remarkable. She did not shut out or withdraw from the world, though at times that seemed like the easiest escape. Instead she chose to open herself up and share her struggle with so many. Her incredible strength gave her the ability to expose her weaknesses to others, which, believe me, was one of the hardest things she was faced with in her lifetime. For those of you who don't know my mother, she was a person who was always giving and, at times, she was annoyingly unselfish. She learned to allow people to take care of her and was able to accept this help. For someone who was so proud and independent, this did not come easy. I can honestly say that caring for my mother was the most rewarding experience of my life, and I am so grateful to her for giving me this opportunity.

I want to share with you all a passage that my mother wrote in her diary shortly after she was diagnosed. "I am learning so much about how many people really respect who I am and how I've lived my life, including people I really respect. I want to fight for time to love and respect what they are responding to in myself, from within myself. [I want] to use that strength and centeredness without question, reserve, or lack of confidence." This reminded me that she was not remarkable for having cancer but for choosing to live as she did with that cancer. She is an example that while we cannot control the amount of time we are given, we do have full control over what we chose to do with the time we have.

Throughout my mother's illness, there were so many people who helped my family in an endless number of ways. Every person was and is appreciated, and their kind gestures meant a great deal. I know that it can be very awkward to approach someone who is dealing with a trauma or who is grieving a loss. People often worry about saying the wrong thing or about not being able to find the perfect words. Well, there are no magic words to take away somebody's pain, but showing your support and telling someone you are there for them, whenever needed, provides a comfort and sense that you will stick by them and share their hard time. This may be exactly what that person needs to hear. All of my friends are and were so wonderful to me, and I am forever grateful to them. If you are ever faced with befriending a person through a difficult time, whether it be cancer or a different challenge, it will help for you to know that it is people's kind gestures and support that are remembered. Though you may not think a person wants you to bring up their situation, it is more important for them to know you are there and will remain present in their life no matter what. My mother would often write about how different people related to her. She wrote about one of her physicians that "he helped me simply by being who he is." I believe that we can all learn from her example. No matter what life brings, there are always choices. My mother has taught me to embrace the challenges that life brings, because good can come from even the toughest of situations.

Tools for Making the System Work for You and Yours

✿ Joan and I spent hundreds of hours gathering information, sorting through treatment options, and communicating with health care providers and insurers. We—like many who have dealt with life-challenging illnesses—developed considerable expertise in navigating the health care system. Appendix B shares some of the more concrete aspects of this expertise, including examples of how we organized and presented information for discussion with health care providers and insurers.

The information presented in the various sections of this appendix is not intended as a guide to dealing with colon cancer. Fortunately the information we gathered and drew upon four, five, and six years ago is now out of date. There are new and more efficacious treatments available now. Avastin, Erbitux, Oxaliplatin, Ironetecan (CPT-11), and Xeloda are now approved by the FDA for various forms of colon cancer. None of these drugs were when Joan was first diagnosed. No doubt the treatment landscape will change again within a couple of years, offering even better options.

Drawing on our experience with colon cancer, appendix B has more general application across other cancers as well as other life-challenging illnesses. The first section of this appendix briefly discusses the types of resources we used to identify treatment choices. The next section presents examples of how we organized information for discussion with health care providers. The third presents several examples of our communications with insurers, and the final section provides some information about how we sought access to experimental treatments.

A couple of words of caution. What we learned about Joan's illness and treatment was beneficial, in large part, because of the mutual respect and generally excellent communication existing between her physicians, other health care providers, and ourselves. Sufficiently secure in their own medical knowledge, her physicians did not resent—and usually welcomed—our questions, the involvement of our friend Dr. George Igel, the information gained from consultations, and, on occasion, an interesting idea gleaned from our own research. For us to have put the kind of information we gathered to best use, we needed to have confidence in Joan's health care providers and work with people who were open to partnering with their patients.

LOCATING USEFUL INFORMATION

When Joan was first diagnosed, I had no idea of how easy it is for laypeople to access relevant health information on the Internet. I began by exploring the Web site of the National Cancer Institute (NCI) (http://www.cancer.gov). NCI's Web site provides access to the most recent research findings and information about the availability of clinical trials concerning treatment for every form of cancer. The clinical trial search engine (http://www.cancer.gov/clinicaltrials) is very powerful, allowing users to search by disease, stage of disease, geographic availability, and enrollment criteria. NCI also has a Cancer Information Service with a toll-free line (1–800–4-CANCER) that provides information in English and Spanish about specific cancers and clinical trials. Additionally, like the other divisions of our National Institutes of Health, NCI also conducts clinical studies on their medical campus. If enrolled in one of these trials, there is no cost to patients for treatment. The transportation and housing costs of patients and a close family member are often paid as well. Information about these NCI trials can be found by calling a toll-free number (1–888-NCI-1937) or by checking their Web site (http://ccr.ncifcrf.gov/triaals/cssc/default.asp).

NCI's Web site also lists information about newly approved cancer treatments (http://www.cancer.gov/clinicaltrials/developments/newly-approved-treatments) and coping with cancer (http://www.cancer.gov/cancertopics/coping). In particular, NCI's Physician Data Query (PDQ) is very useful. The PDQ is regularly updated by experts and summarizes the state of the art for each of roughly 110 adult cancers and 50 childhood cancers. This information is presented in two versions—for patients/family members and for health care providers:

> PDQ (Physician Data Query) is NCI's comprehensive cancer database. It contains peer reviewed summaries on cancer treatment, screening, prevention, genetics, and supportive care, and complementary and alternative medicine; a registry of approximately 2,000 open and 13,000 closed cancer clinical trials from around the world; and directories of physicians, professionals who provide genetics services, and organizations that provide cancer care.
>
> PDQ contains evidence-based summaries that provide prognostic and treatment information on the major types of cancer in adults [and children]. . . . The PDQ adult [and child] treatment summaries are also available in patient versions, written in easy-to-understand, non-technical language. (Accessed on August 9, 2004, from the NCI Web site, http://www.cancer.gov/cancertopics/pdq/cancerdatabase#summaries)

For someone needing an accurate overview of the state of the knowledge and treatment of specific cancers, the PDQ treatment summaries are the best place to begin. This information can be accessed at http://www.cancer.gov/cancerinfo/pdq/adulttreatment and http://www.cancer.gov/cancerinfo/pdq/pediatrictreatment.

In early October 1998, Dr. Lionel Rudolph suggested looking at the availability of clinical trials and provided me with abstracts of research papers about CPT-11 and Oxaliplatin, two drugs that later benefited Joan. He had downloaded these abstracts for us from Medline (http://www.nlm.nih.gov/portals/healthcare.html), the online cata-logue of the National Institutes of Health's National Library of Medicine.

Medline provides access to 14 million biomedical research citations and in many cases short summaries of findings (abstracts) going back fifty years (http://www.ncbi.nlm.nih.gov/entrez/query.fcgi). The full text of some articles can also be accessed, if you are so inclined. Informa-tion about the availability of clinical trials can also be found on this Web site (http://clinicaltrials.gov/).

There are many other excellent sources of information as well. Pro-fessional organizations publish the programs and abstracts of recent meetings where the latest scientific findings are presented. Many also provide access to their journals, either abstracts of full-text articles or links to relevant public and private organizations. The Web site of the American Society of Clinical Oncology (ASCO) is particularly useful (http://www.asco.org). The Web sites of organizations like the Ameri-can Cancer Society (http://www.cancer.org) are sources of information about treatment options or where to go to find information about virtu-ally anything in the cancer world, from clinical trials to support groups, from statistics to wigs. Similarly, disease-specific advocacy groups such as the Colon Cancer Alliance (http://www.ccalliance.org) can provide excellent up-to-date information about treatment choices, access to sup-port services, volunteer opportunities, and ways of communicating your interests to legislators, administrative bodies, and the press.

The Web sites of major cancer centers such as Memorial Sloan-Kettering Cancer Center (http://www.mskcc.org) and M. D. Anderson Cancer Center (http://www.mdanderson.org) also serve as points of access to the types of information already described. These Web sites also provide information about research protocols and treating physi-cians at their centers. Similarly, other specialized centers such as the Jay Monahan Center for Gastrointestinal Health at the New York Presbyter-ian Hospital (http://www.monahancenter.org) and Cornell's Weill Medical College serve as sources for information and care of selected ill-nesses as may other local and regional hospitals.

The Association of Cancer Online Resources (ACOR; http://

www.acor.org) is another excellent source of support and online information. It provides links to chat groups, listservs, and other sources of support for disease-specific and more general (ostomy, pain control) concerns. Listservs should be approached with the understanding that not all of the information provided is accurate.

Combined with what we were learning from the doctors and our own research, I found one of Yahoo's colon cancer listservs very helpful (http://health.groups.yahoo.com/group/colon_cancer_support). When Joan was considering surgery for interperitoneal tumors, I sent a message to the listserv inquiring whether others had gone through the surgery. Several people identified themselves and offered to speak with Joan, offers Joan accepted and found quite useful. When we needed to locate a surgeon, we cross-checked the names of people we had been given by our physicians with the experiences of several people on the listserv. It helped confirm that, given Joan's concern to maintain quality of life, one particularly aggressive surgical approach was not for her. Reading daily through the posts, I often found information that helped me "reality check" whether we might be overlooking some important avenue, whether Joan's reactions to the chemo were similar to others on similar protocols, etc. There were a couple of scientifically knowledgeable persons on the list who shared their views about the promise of certain trials. And there were some people whose humanity and concerns for others, while in the midst of their own struggles, was comforting.

My experience is that medical and pharmacological researchers and personnel are willing to provide information when asked. Although they are extremely busy, most responded graciously to our telephone calls, e-mails, letters, and faxes. One helpfully steered us away from participating in a trial of a drug that was eventually withdrawn as a viable treatment option. Another "medical stranger" arranged for Joan's tumor to be assessed in terms of potential efficacy of treatment by selected chemotherapies.

The information we gathered from many sources was very helpful. However, at times it was also disturbing and frightening. Reading about the short survival prospects of people in Joan's situation was not what I wanted to learn. I told myself that the very poor outcomes were generally based on studies begun five to ten years earlier, but still it would have been much better to learn that her odds were good. The potential to misread or fail to understand the meaning of information gathered is great, especially for people like me who are not trained in the biomedical sciences. And so, I cautioned myself and would caution others to be careful about jumping to any conclusions.

Then there is the good old-fashioned way of collecting information: books. Take a browse through the health/self-help section of a large bookstore or go to the public library.

Below are three examples of information I accessed on the Internet when I was researching treatment choices in 1998 and 1999:

"SURGICAL TREATMENT OF COLORECTAL METASTASES TO THE LIVER"

Y. Fong, L. H. Blumgart, and A. M. Cohen. *CA: Cancer Journal for Clinicians* 45, no. 1 (Jan.–Feb. 1995): 50–62. PMID 7804899.
Department of Surgery, Memorial Sloan-Kettering Cancer Center, New York, N.Y.

Up to one fourth of patients diagnosed with colorectal cancer present with liver metastases, and by the time of death, up to 70 percent of patients with colorectal cancer have metastatic disease to the liver. At present, surgical excision is the standard therapy for resectable liver metastases from colorectal primaries. This article reviews the natural history of colorectal metastases to the liver and results of studies of systemic chemotherapy, surgical resection, and alternative surgical approaches.

"TREATMENT OF COLORECTAL CANCER: HEPATIC METASTASIS"

Y. Fong, N. Kemeny, P. Paty, L. H. Blumgart, and A. M. Cohen. *Seminars in Surgical Oncology* 12, no. 4 (July–Aug. 1996): 219–52. Review. PMID: 8829283.

Colorectal Service, Department of Surgery, Gastrointestinal
Oncology Service, Memorial Sloan-Kettering Cancer
Center, New York, N.Y.

Almost one-third of patients dying from colorectal cancer
have tumors limited to the liver. Systemic chemotherapy is the
appropriate palliative management of patients with metastases
to the liver and other sites. For many patients with isolated
hepatic metastases, systemic chemotherapy is also the most
appropriate treatment. However, results with systemic chemotherapy indicate that one-third or less of patients will respond to such treatments, and long-term survival is rare. In this
report we provide information concerning the natural history
of colorectal hepatic metastases, followed by the expected benefits with systemic chemotherapy. This information provides
background for the regional therapeutic strategies of surgical
resection, cryosurgery, and hepatic artery chemotherapy. We
discuss the selection factors appropriate for such treatments,
morbidity and mortality, and the potential long-term benefits of
such approaches. The last section focuses on surgical considera-
tions in hepatic resection and hepatic artery chemotherapy.

"HEPATIC ARTERIAL INFUSION OF CHEMOTHERAPY AFTER RESECTION OF HEPATIC METASTASES FROM COLORECTAL CANCER"

Nancy Kemeny, Ying Huang, Alfred M. Cohen, Weiji Shi, John
A. Conti, Murray F. Brennan, Joseph R. Bertino, Alan D. M.
Turnbull, Deirdre Sullivan, Jennifer Stockman, Leslie H.
Blumgart, and Yuman Fong. *New England Journal of
Medicine* 341 (1999): 2039–48.

Abstract

Background. Two years after undergoing resection of liver
metastases from colorectal cancer, about 65 percent of patients

are alive and 25 percent are free of detectable disease. We tried to improve these outcomes by treating patients with hepatic arterial infusion of floxuridine plus systemic fluorouracil after liver resection.

Methods. We randomly assigned 156 patients at the time of resection of hepatic metastases from colorectal cancer to receive six cycles of hepatic arterial infusion with floxuridine and dexamethasone plus intravenous fluorouracil, with or without leucovorin, or six weeks of similar systemic therapy alone. Patients were stratified according to previous treatment and the number of liver metastases identified at operation. The study end points were overall survival, survival without recurrence of hepatic metastases, and survival without any metastases at two years.

Results. The actuarial rate of overall survival at two years was 86 percent in the group treated with combined therapy and 72 percent in the group given monotherapy alone ($P = 0.03$). The median survival was 72.2 months in the combined-therapy group and 59.3 months in the monotherapy group, with a median follow-up of 62.7 months. After two years, the rates of survival free of hepatic recurrence were 90 percent in the combined-therapy group and 60 percent in the monotherapy group ($P < 0.001$), and the respective rates of progression-free survival were 57 percent and 42 percent ($P = 0.07$). At two years, the risk ratio for death was 2.34 among patients treated with systemic therapy alone, as compared with patients who received combined therapy (95 percent confidence interval, 1.10 to 4.98; $P = 0.027$), after adjustment for important variables. The rates of adverse effects of at least moderate severity were similar in the two groups, except for a higher frequency of diarrhea and hepatic effects in the combined-therapy group.

Conclusions. For patients who undergo resection of liver metastases from colorectal cancer, postoperative treatment with a combination of hepatic arterial infusion of floxuridine and intravenous fluorouracil improves the outcome at two years.

KEEPING TREATMENT NOTES

Option Memos for Doctors

In the midst of diagnosis and at those junctures where major decisions need to be made about the course of treatment, it is important to take good notes of your discussions with your doctors. It's also helpful to have an extra set of ears present for these discussions. People sometimes think they will remember everything, but our experience was that there was much we forgot. Included below are two examples of some of the notes we took. The first is from two discussions with Joan's gastroenterologist, one right after he discovered a mass in Joan's colon during her September 1998 colonoscopy and the second when the biopsy results came back. The second summarizes advice given informally by two physicians, Dr. Lionel Rudolph, the husband of a colleague, and Dr. George Igel, a close friend.

With the exception of a few minor changes, in this section and those that follow, the emphasis, spelling, and format have been left as they were in the original documents.

ERIC'S NOTES: DISCUSSION WITH DR. MARK KASOWITZ
(after colonoscope—9/24/98)

Something in right colon
    Multi-lobulated mass in right colon near cecum
    Villus Adenoma—looks like a polyp that has been around
        for a long time
    about 4–5 centimeters
    at base of cecum
Also a small polyp but no reason to do anything with it today
    as it will be taken care of when you take care of larger one
Biopsied tissue and will contact with results
Recommends surgery—Wants to set up appointment with Dr.
    Brown
Will take off entire right colon and rejoin to ileum. Ileum will
    be attached to transverse colon

Nothing on CT scan that suggests liver or lymph spread of
  cancer
Lab work o.k., too. Even though lab work came back negative,
  his experience suggests it may be cancerous
Laproscopic surgery not recommended—could do right colon
  resection with lap, but only shortens recovery by a couple
  of days
Colostomy will not be needed
If benign or non-invasive—no chemo
If spread, 5FU most likely

ERIC'S NOTES: OTHER SEPTEMBER 1998 DISCUSSIONS

Advice from Dr. Lionel Rudolph

Mentioned Dr. K's referral to Dennis Brown and said he would
  be excellent
Recommends Dr. X at Crouse for anesthesia
Make your concerns about anesthesia very clear
Pretty standard surgery for a good surgeon. Recovery quick
If there is a question about malignancy and chemo, ask that an
  oncologist be brought in to give a nonsurgical opinion
  about how to treat malignancy

Advice from Dr. George Igel

Make clear of the type of thyroid problem you had—a
  follicular adenoma
Make clear that only Dr. Brown operates
Think about what the recuperative stage will be like—expect 2
  or 3 month recuperation

Treatment History

Our friend George encouraged us to keep a running history of treatments and major test results so that we could provide health care
providers with a quick precis of Joan's illness. To facilitate communica-

tion among her physicians, we also added names and contact information of her treating physicians. This was extremely helpful, particularly when we needed to contact new physicians. I have included, as prepared primarily by Joan, her treatment history through May 2000. The telephone numbers and health insurance identification numbers have been altered to preserve confidentiality.

TREATMENT HISTORY OF JOAN KINGSON

8278 Glen Eagle Drive, Manlius, NY 13104
315-682-xxxx (H) 315-430-xxxx (cell) E-mail: Kingson@xxx

Health Insurance: Blue Cross Blue Shield of Central New York.
   Telephone #s 315-448-xxxx 800-479-xxxx. Identification #
   SYU087xx xxxx-02. Group # 64 xxxx. BS Plan Code xxx BC
   Plan Code xxx
Social Security #: 117-xx-xxxx

Treating Physicians

Dr. Nancy Kemeny—primary oncologist. Her address is Memorial Sloan-Kettering Hospital, 1275 York Avenue, New York, NY 10021. 212-639-xxxx. Her nurse, Karen Ragusa, can be reached at 212-610-xxxx.

Dr. Anthony Scalzo—Syracuse-based oncologist and coordinates care with Dr. Nancy Kemeny. Dr. Scalzo's address is Hematology-Oncology, 1000 East Genesee St., Suite 400, Syracuse, NY 13210. 315-472-xxxx.

Dr. Yuman Fong is the surgeon who performed the liver resection and implantation of HAI pump at Memorial Sloan-Kettering. His telephone number is 212-639-xxxx.

Dr. Dennis Brown is the surgeon who performed the hemicolectomy in Syracuse. His telephone numbers are 315-492-xxxx, 470-xxxx, 492-xxxx.

Primary care and annual physical exams—Dr. Paul Kronenberg. His office serves as the gatekeeper for referrals. 739 Irving Avenue, Syracuse, NY 13210. 315-479-xxxx.

Gyn—Dr. Susan Nitka. I see her for regular pelvic exams, pap smears, and mammograms. 315-474-xxxx.

Hospitalization prior to 1998

July 1996. Surgery (thyroidectomy) Pathology report— Right total, left subtotal thyroidectomy, follicular adenoma (3.5 cm). Benign.

History Related to Colon Cancer

January 1998. Initial symptoms. Isolated incident of asymptomatic bloody stool.

May–August 1998. Intermittent episodes of abdominal pain increasing in intensity and frequency throughout this period.

September 1998. Moved to Syracuse, New York, entered local health care system, began month long period of testing including a barium enema and completed colonoscopy (both revealed a mass at the ileal-cecal valve). Mass biopsied. Pathology inconclusive.

October 1998. Hemi-colectomy performed at Syracuse's Crouse Hospital. Pathology report revealed adenocarcinoma with involvement of seven out of thirty lymph nodes taken. CT scan later that week revealed metastases in the liver.

November 1998. Consultation with Dr. Robert Mayer, Dana Farber Cancer Institute. Consultation with Dr. Nancy Kemeny, Sloan-Kettering Cancer Center. Decision to work with Dr. Kemeny whose recommended approach was more aggressive and immediate.

December 1998. Underwent surgery with Dr. Yuman Fong at Sloan: liver resection and implantation of hepatic pump through biliary artery (mesenteric artery bifurcates before the liver, therefore not an option for catheter implantation). Recovered from surgery quickly and well—began regular walks of a couple miles approximately twelve days post-op.

January 1999. Began six-month course of systemic CPT-11 and FUDR directly to liver from pump. Morbidity included temporary digestive discomfort and some back pain on right side. These symptoms resolved by July 1999. Protocol required follow-up CT scans every three months. These were clear until October 1999.

October 1999. CT scan identified "suspicious findings" in the abdomen—confirmed by needle-guided biopsy to be disease consistent with the primary tumor.

November 1999. Met with Dr. Kemeny who ordered PET scan. Based on results of this test, she recommended protocol of oxaliplatin and CPT-11 to be delivered systematically (four weeks in a cycle, followed by two weeks off). Her goal was to produce sufficient shrinkage for surgical resection and peritoneal wash.

November–March 1999. Have tolerated protocol very well with few side effects. Weight loss has been minimal, chemistries are close to normal range, and have maintained routine daily exercise of walking two to three miles daily.

February 2, 2000. CT scan shows no indication of previously visible nodules soft tissue densities in omentum and the mesentery.

February 28, 2000. PET scan shows that "compared to previous exam of November 2, 1999, there has been a marked reduction in the number of areas of hypermetabolism. . . . Overall, there has been a significant reduction in the size and metabolism of the lesions within the abdomen and pelvis and in areas the maximal SUV is reduced." Reviewing this scan, Dr. Kemeny recommended seeking surgical resection with peritoneal wash.

March 2000. Consulted with Dr. Brian Loggie in Winston-Salem, N.C. Currently moving practice to Texas. After reviewing reports and scans and consulting with Dr. Kemeny, he indicated that abdominal surgery with chemotherapeutic wash could be planned for June in Texas. Recommended minimally four weeks off chemotherapy prior to surgery and immediate trial with 5 FU because CEA rising. (This became my third chemotherapy protocol).

April 2000. Met with Dr. Kemeny. Prescribed course of Xeloda (4000 mg daily, initially two weeks on, one week off; now one week on, one off) combined with Celebrex (400 mg daily) prior to surgery in June. Could not maintain initial two/one-week arrangement due to blisters and lowering of platelets to 70 so switched to one/one after being off Xeloda for two weeks. CEA went from 14 to 21 during the two-week hiatus.

April 7, 2000. CT scan to be used as baseline for efficacy of Xeloda. Showed minimal change from previous CT scan.

Late April to May 2000. Moderate rise in CEA (from 8 to 21) since going off Oxaliplatin.

April 25, 2000. Identified probable metastasis on scar line below stomach. Palpable node on left side of scar line.

May 2000. Negative mammogram. Pap smear indicated questionable cells. Follow-up colposcopy was negative.

May 24, 2000. PET scan of higher resolution (at Sloan) than the February and November PET scans (at private setting) indicated some increase in disease in the abdominal cavity and very small spot in the liver. New clinical symptom of "foot-drop" in the right foot reported to Dr. Kemeny. Follow-up MRI scheduled for June 1 and neurological exam scheduled for June 6.

Planning in Advance for Appointments

George also encouraged us to organize carefully information we wanted to report and questions we wanted to ask in advance of key meetings with physicians, again, advice that was extremely helpful. We often went over these questions in great detail with George and developed several drafts. Insofar as possible, we tried to get our key questions on one page. Whenever possible, we faxed this information in advance of meeting with physicians and nurses. We also gave a copy of this information to the health care providers present when Joan had her office visits. To foster communication among health care providers and take advantage of their expertise, we also communicated concerns in short letters.

Following in this section are several examples of the information we provided physicians. The first presents list of questions at our initial meeting (November 11, 1998) with Dr. Kemeny. We broke the brevity rule on this one. Even so, we separated our major questions from the long list of possible interventions we had identified through our research. I believe we gave Dr. Kemeny the questions at the beginning of the office visit. Toward the end of the visit, we gave her the list of possible interventions, and she went through this list and identified the ones that might be worth considering at some point. We kept this list of possible interventions and, over the thirty-two-month period, added to it as we identified new interventions. (Again, I have included the information as we presented it, spelling errors and all.)

The second example is an October 23, 1999, letter to Dr. Yuman Fong, Joan's surgeon at Sloan. This was sent after a CT scan suggested her tumor had spread to the peritoneal cavity and in advance of a needle biopsy.

The third is a list of questions for Dr. Kemeny for a February 23, 2000, office visit to assess whether Joan's peritoneal tumors were responding to chemotherapy (Oxaliplatin/CPT-11). The fourth is a list of questions from April 5, 2000, for Dr. Kemeny about issues related to surgery to remove tumors in the peritoneal cavity. (Names of the surgeons we were considering have been removed.)

The fifth is a set of questions we faxed on June 14, 2000, to Dr. Richard Swanson's nurse-practitioner, Mary Ryan, in advance of Joan's surgery with Dr. Swanson. The sixth is a list of questions we prepared for Dr. Swanson and his team in advance of Joan's July 2000 surgery.

Trying to stay one step ahead of the cancer, we sent a July 11, 2000, letter, the seventh example, to Dr. Kemeny—with a list of possible interventions—requesting her advice about postsurgical treatments to consider after Dr. Swanson's surgery. Also, a September 24, 2000, letter to Dr. Kemeny was sent in advance of a scheduled October surgery that was later canceled because Joan's cancer had spread. This letter also lays out questions about follow-up treatments.

Lists of Questions and of Possible Interventions for First Meeting with Dr. Nancy Kemeny
November 11, 1998

Here are the questions we hope to answer prior to beginning treatment:

Which current treatment currently offers the greatest response?

Are there any developing treatments (e.g., new drug, new approach or clinical trials) that we should consider? Risks?

What can be added to the treatment (e.g., Tomudex, oxaliplatin, interferon, Rebif, CPT-11, Farnecine Transferase) to improve outcomes? Risks?

Is hyperthermia something that should be considered? Under what circumstances? In conjunction with other therapies?

Do you agree with the recommendation that we should wait several months? Are there any interventions that should be considered in the interim?

Might a tumor vaccine be something to pursue (e.g., reference to New Yorker article) What's your reaction to the use of large quantities of SPES (Chinese herb referenced in New Yorker article)? Is there a way to tell whether Joan's cancer has a p53 mutation?

What combinations of interventions should be considered (e.g., cryosurgery, infusion, followed by 5FU???)? Risks?

What are the quality of life issues? What is the rhythm of various protocols? How do people tolerate the protocols? Range of responses among individuals? Side effects?

Are there investigational programs being offered at Sloan Farber, Roswell, elsewhere that we should consider?

Can the metastases be removed by surgery by someone who is an aggressive cancer surgeon? Should some type of less invasive surgery be considered (e.g., cryosurgery). Some type of ablation (e.g., alcohol). Radiation? Heat?

Should we start by going after the liver first and then consider more systemic treatment?

Can (should) the recommended therapy be done in Syracuse?

Are there any other things we need to know about the state of this cancer before beginning treatment? Are more tests needed?

How will we know if something is working? Not working? How long?

How does your practice work? How can, should this be coordinated with Dr. Scalzo and Dr. Brown?

How to prepare for treatment? Flu shots, Pneumonia vaccine, types of food, storing own blood? Vitamins? Nutrition supplement?

Are there supportive therapies we should explore? Ones that can't hurt and may help (e.g. massage. acupuncture, aspirin, vitamins, herbs, holistic approaches)?

Here are the various interventions we have come across. Which ones might hold promise for us?

Tomudex—New drug understudy at Sloan. Told that there have been some cases of complete remission

Oxaloplatin—(Think this drug is in use in France)—"Synergistic effects with traditional therapy 5FU/folonic acid have increased response rates significantly, improved time sensitive parameters and facilitated the removal of previously unresectable hepatic metastases" (Ducreaux M, Louvet C, Bekradda, M & Cvitkovic E, Service de Gastroenterologie et d'Oncologie Digestive, Institut Gustave, Roussy, Villejuif, France, Semin Oncol; 25(2 Suppl 5): 47–53 1998)

Rebif (recombinant interferon gamma)—new drug in phase III study in 1998. Manufactured by Serono Labs in Norwell, Massachusetts

Marminastat

Farnacine transferase

Hyperthermia—whole body or selective

Sulinduc

Artery infusion (HAI) of interleukin-2-based immunochemo-therapy—Article presents "cases of three patients with multiple liver metastases from colorectal cancer in whom complete remission was achieved by treatment with HAI of IL-2 in combination with mitomycin C (MMC) and 5-FU" (Okuno K, Ohnishi, H; Nakajima, I; Akabane, Y; Kurooka, K, Koh, K, Shindo K & Yasutomi M—First Dept of Surgery, Kinki University, School of Medicine, Osaka, Japan, Surg Today, 24 (1): 80–84 1994).

Surgical resection (or bypass of obstructing primary lesion)

Surgical resection of isolated metastases

Tumor vaccine—Dr. Eli Gilboa at Duke University is testing different types of tumor vaccines for bowel cancer

Radiotheraphy

5FU & Leukovorin

Cryosurgery

Embolization—(explained as catheterizing the hepatic artery and throwing in tiny particles to kill the cancers)

Interstitial radiotherapy—(Think this involves delivering radioactive material to site of metastases)

Arterial infusion

Combining interarterial chemo with hepatic irradiation

Oral 5FU—in phases II and phase III trials

5FU with methotrixate

CPT-11 (may be called Ironitecan, Camptusar)—new colon cancer drug that has been effective when cancer not responsive to 5FU

Vascular targeting agents (not sure what this means)

High dose of perfusion with TNF (Tumor Necrosis Factor)—Dr. Douglas Fraker at Penn. In clinical phase II trial for patients with liver only disease

1 hour recirculating perfusion of vascularly isolated liver (IHP). Mitomycin C and melaphalan entered phase 1 and 2 trials on IHP. (Vahrmeijer AL, Van Der Eb MM, Van Dierendock, JH &

Kuppen, PJ, Dept. of Surgery, Leiden University Medical
Center, The Netherlands, Simin Surg Oncol 14(3): 262–68
1998)

Letter to Dr. Yuman Fong before an Appointment
to Address CT Scan Results
October 23, 1999

Joan F. Kingson
8278 Glen Eagle Drive
Manlius, NY 13104

Dr. Yuman Fong
Hepatobiliary Service
Department of Surgery
Memorial Sloan-Kettering Cancer Center
1275 York Avenue
New York, NY 10021

Dear Dr. Fong,

Last Thursday (10/21) I had my three month follow-up CT
scan and chest x-ray (please see enclosed films and attached
written reports). The findings are suspicious of a recurrence and
an ultra-sound guided needle biopsy has been scheduled to
take place at Crouse Hospital here in Syracuse on Tuesday
morning (10/26). I believe the area to be biopsied is close to the
catheter entering the liver from my hepatic pump.

Would you kindly review these films and reports. We have
three questions—Is there anything that the physician performing this procedure should be especially aware of in relation to
the catheter? As you will recall my catheter is unusually small
and was placed in the biliary artery. Is there anything special
that should be communicated to this person? Any advice or im-
pressions from the scan that you might have for us would be
very much appreciated. Eric and I can be reached at 315-682-
xxxx (home) or 315-243-xxxx (cell phone).

Our next appointment is scheduled with Dr. Kemeny for Wednesday November 3.

Thank you for taking the time to respond to this request.

Sincerely,

Joan F. Kingson

Questions for an Appointment with Dr. Kemeny Discussing the Efficacy of the Current Treatment
February 23, 2000

What does the recent CT scan mean? Does it alter your view with regard to possible surgery and possible peritoneal wash?

How do you evaluate continued success of chemo?

Is the goal to bring the CEA down more?

Should I have a PET scan?

Is there a possibility of doing one or two treatments in a cycle in Syracuse?

In an article I saw that the average amount of time on Oxaliplatin without a relapse is about 20 weeks. Given this, is there a point at which it would be appropriate to consider adding additional approaches (e.g., anti-angiogenesis, monoclonal antibodies, ???)?

Is there any way to treat the extreme sensitivity to cold that follows the chemo? Can this result in permanent damage? Are hand-warmers a useful way to treat this? (Have Joan describe)

Are headaches a side effect of Neupogen? I seem to get them after two days of taking Neupogen.

Sensations—Left back, near kidney; sometimes sensations at the pelvic floor.

Any diagnostic significance to the kidney being out of normal position?

Veins—I understand rationale for not getting a port, but my experience is that this chemo is very caustic and my vein hurt up to 4 or 5 days after infusion. Is there anything that can be done to make the infusion and the aftermath less painful?

What is the current Alk Phos and why is it remaining slightly elevated? How long should I continue to take the Actigal

What type of white blood cell count do you want me to maintain between treatment?

What data do you want to be sure to have when we come to visit you? CEA?

Need pump refilled

Need Neupogen

Thanks, much

Questions to Presurgical Appointment with Dr. Kemeny
April 5, 2000

What do you think about Dr. X's recommendations? Would you recommend using 5FU? Would this be, with or without, Leucovoran? Alternatively, might Xeloda be used to preserve veins?

Can we receive the treatment locally? What would the plan be?

What are the possible side effects of 5FU?

Do we know whether Joan's tumor has high levels of enzyme thymidylate synthase (TS) and/or DPD? We've seen reference to research on pilot studies that indicate when measuring these two enzymes, TS and DPD, if the patient is 1. above the threshold of either or both—no response to 5-FU; 2. below the threshold of both—most will respond; 3) much toxicity if two mutant genes result in very high DPD

Would you update Dr. Scalzo (315-472-xxxx) and discuss the plan with him?

What do you make of the rise in CEA?

What do you make of the moderate rise in liver enzymes? Could it be a result of the chemo therapy? Are you seeing this with other people in the CPT-11/Oxaliplatin protocol?

Dr. X suggested taking vitamins A, C and E in preparation for surgery? What do you think? Vitamin C has been in the news recently as something colon cancer patients should avoid?

We're not sure how long I should be off chemo therapy in preparation for surgery? If I go on 5FU, would 4 weeks be sufficient?

Should I think about banking blood?

Should we schedule a PET scan? CT scan?

We got the impression that Dr. X may have been concerned about my being on Neupogen? Should I try to be off of it in advance of surgery?

Here are Dr. X's telephone numbers:

Need pump refilled

Need Neupogen

What are your recommendations about contacts with other surgeons? We are very comfortable with Dr. X and his approach, if you are. Should we keep April 24 appointment with Dr. Y? For now, it does seem to make sense to keep the appointment with Dr. Z.

Pre-Op Questions for the Nurse-Practitioner Assisting
with Upcoming Surgery
June 14, 2000

Dear Mary,

Can't say that we're exactly looking forward to our stay in Worcester, but we are pleased that it will be with Dr. Swanson and you.

We are sending these questions to you anticipating that it may be helpful for you to have them in advance of our conversation.

1. *Additional Tests*—PET Scan—Does Dr. Swanson need any more information from scans prior to surgery? If another PET

scan is needed, would it be preferable that it be done on the same machine at Sloan? If so, we'll need some time to set this up. CT Scan—Would you like us to send the latest (April 7) CT scan films? Would you like another CT? MRI?

2. *Vaccines before surgery*—Dr. Swanson mentioned that there were three vaccines that I should get in advance of surgery just in case there is a need to remove the spleen? What are the vaccines? How should I proceed with this? Timing?

3. *Reversible ostomy*—If an ostomy is needed, I would prefer—if at all possible—that it be reversible. Is this something that needs to be thought about in advance of surgery? Are there any downsides to a reversible as opposed to a nonreversible ostomy?

4. *Banking Blood*—Should I ask my sister (same blood type) to bank blood for me? She could bank it in Worcester.

5. *Pump*—Given the heated wash, is it important that the pump be filled with glycerin before and immediately after the surgery? Should Dr. Swanson have contact with Medtronics? Also, because this pump is placed in the biliary vein, might it be important to get the smaller tubing that the company sent to Dr. Fong to connect it to this vein? Should Dr. Swanson be in contact with Dr. Fong?

6. *Tumor samples*—Can we plan to preserve as large a tumor sample as possible? Should part of the sample be frozen and do they have this ability? Is there any other information we could get from the tumor to further target treatments? Are there some special assays that should be considered? If so, do we need to get some of this in place in advance of surgery?

I've been in contact with Dr. Kemeny about stopping chemo. She indicates I should go off Celebrex 10 days before surgery. She'll watch my blood work and make a decision about the Xeloda. June 5 blood work (CEA = 18.5. WBC = 4.8; PLT = 130;

RBC = 3.1; HGB = 11.4); June 12 blood work (CEA = 21.4. WBC = 4.5; PLT = 1151; RBC = 2.95; HGB = 11.1)

Thanks,

Joan and Eric Kingson 315-682-xxxx (home) 315-430-xxxx (cell)

Questions for Dr. Swanson's Team before Surgery

Effects of Mitomycin C

If there is a reaction, when is it likely to occur? What should I look for?

How often should I have blood drawn during the next two weeks? After that? If there is a chemo-related problem, who should deal with it? Dr. Swanson? Dr. Kemeny? Dr. Scalzo—oncologist in Syracuse)?

Pathology Report

Does the pathology report indicate whether the tumors were from the primary tumor?

Have there been any pathology studies that provide additional information about the tumor (e.g., are the TS levels high?) that we should know about?

Is there anything else about the tumor that you may have learned in surgery that would be useful for us to know? Were they able to freeze some of the tumor?

CEA

Has a CEA been taken since surgery? What is it?

Restrictions and Exercises

What are the major restrictions? Diet? Climbing stairs? Lifting?

Conversely, any movements or exercises I should be trying to do?

Questions on Hysterectomy

Do I still have a cervix?

What, if anything, should I think about in terms of the effects of being without ovaries and uterus?

When might we safely resume sexual relations? What, if anything, should we be aware of?

Follow-up

When would you like to see me? How regularly?

When should the staples come out?

Have you had a discussion with Dr. Kemeny about follow-up and continued treatment?

Any treatment recommendations, experimental or otherwise?

Reversing the Ileostomy

While I do not feel there is any rush to reverse the ileostomy, we are wondering whether there might be any benefit to doing a prophylactic wash (e.g., misogynic, fur) when you reverse it? Might periodic laproscopic washes be of any benefit?

What Tests Are Best to Monitor the Illness?

CT? PET? MRI? CEA? Various tests tumor sample?

Copies of Reports

Would you send copies of the CT, surgical and path reports to Dr. Nancy Kemeny (Memorial Sloan-Kettering Cancer Center, 1275 York Avenue, New York, NY 10021, fax 212-717-xxxx) and Dr. Anthony Scalzo (Hematology-Oncology Associates, 1000 East Genesee St., Suite 400, Syracuse, NY 13210, Fax 508-479-xxxx). May we have copies of the CT, surgical and path reports? (Joan Kingson, 8278 Glen Eagle Drive, Manlius, NY 13104)

Questions for Dr. Kemeny about Treatment Options after Surgery
July 11, 2000

Dear Dr. Kemeny,

We had a good meeting with Dr. Swanson and the surgery is scheduled for July 17. He indicated that he spoke with you prior to our meeting. Thank you for taking the time to review Joan's situation with him. We are very appreciative of the time you have given to overseeing Joan's care.

Would you mind helping us think through the post-surgical treatment options? We have listed some below and placed asterisks by the ones that are phase III studies or otherwise strike us (as lay persons) as most promising.

Please let us know if you think there are treatment options that might be especially promising—even if it seems that the drug is not available. If need be, our friend, Dr. George Igel, and Eric as well as some of other friends, would be willing to see if gaining access through compassionate use is feasible. Since this might take some time to accomplish, it is probably best that we begin working on this fairly soon.

As we read the list of options, the most immediately feasible/promising ones may be to seek participation in Dr. Welt's study or in Dr. Foon's study (if he is able to gain access to Interleukin 2 to continue this study). Dr. Bilchik's study seems like a possibility, but the logistics would be very difficult and we would appreciate knowing whether you think it is worth putting our energy into this or something else).

In short, your advice would be very welcomed, including suggestions for anything we may have overlooked.

Thanks,

Eric and Joan Kingson

315-682-xxxx home; 315-430-xxxx phone

Possible Interventions

VACCINES

CEA VAC vaccine combined with Interleukin 2—Dr. Foon (513-584-xxxx) has a trial that has begun, but is unable to add more patients because the pharmaceutical company that supplies Interleukin 2 is not providing the drug. There is a reasonable chance that Joan could be eligible for this study after her surgery. CEA VAC (Titan Pharmaceuticals—650-244-xxxx) is going into a phase III study sponsored by the National Cancer Institute and run by the American College of Surgeons Oncology Group. However, Joan is not eligible for this. Seems like best bet is to see whether Joan could enter CEA VAC/Interleukin 2 trial)

Avicenna Vaccine—BIOPHARMA, INC. (Nasdaq:AVII, AVIIW, AVIIZ), multicenter phase III trial for colorectal cancer starting in 2000

CancerVax—Dr. Anton Bilchik—John Wayne Medical Center— requires trips to California every two weeks for several months, then once a month for a year, then somewhat less frequently—Could do, but would want to know if it made sense to do Maria Gonzalez—coordinator—310-449-xxxx (449-xxxx fax)

Dr. Fong's study

CEA-Cide (Immunomedics 973-605-xxxx)—humanized anti-body against CEA. Phase II study

Trials at New York Hospital (Dr. Karen Green—212-746-xxxx)— CEA CIDE by itself

New Jersey Trial CEA CUDE radiolabeled with iodine-131—Dr. George Hajjar and Dr. Malik Juweid—973-844-xxxx

Antibody 105AD7 vaccine—Dr Andrew D. Sutton, Head of Research and Development at Onyvax, Inc. First trials have been initiated in early- and late-stage colorectal cancer patients

MONOCLONAL ANTIBODIES

Dr. Welt's studies—Joan is not eligible for the one for which her tumor was tested. However, she may be eligible (if bilirubin goes down) for the other study that he mentioned (I believe this involves a chemo that tries to boost the immune system, followed by a chemo cocktail that Dr. Kemeny put together *(Carmustine, 5FU, Vincristine & Streptozoci ????)*

C-225—Cetuximab—Imclone Dr. Harlan Waksal—head of research 908-218-xxxx 646-638-xxxx
mille van ness, clinical coordinator 908-541-xxxx
17–1A www.immuogen.

ANTIANGIOGENESIS

Angiostatin—Entremed, Inc.—New trial beginning
SU5416—Maybe useful if we could gain compassionate use of SU5416 and combine with other chemotherapy
SU6668—Joan is on list for SU6668 phase 1 trial—However, it is only being given by itself.
Thalidomide
Tetrathiomolybdate, or TM, copper lowering drug—University of Michigan George J. Brewer, & Sofia Merajver

OTHER OPTIONS—NOT SURE HOW TO CLASSIFY

rhuMAb-VEGF, or anti-VEGF, in combination with chemotherapy—Genentech, Inc.—Susan D. Hellmann, M.D., M.P.H., Genentech's chief medical officer/*Planning phase III trial*—Physicians and people with colorectal cancer interested in anti-VEGF clinical trials should call 1-888-662-xxxx.
Raltitrexed (ICI D1694) and 5FU at MSK (Dr. Schwartz)
IM682 (Cytran) Phase 1 trial. Delivers P53 gene in a viral vector ???
Aptosyn (APC)—triggers APOPTOSIS—Cell Pathways Inc., a Horsham, www.cellpathways.com Think it is associated with Dr. John Marshall at Georgetown
Briostatin—John Marshall Georgetown Sea moss that potntiates other chemos Genetics Professor SCH66336 created by the Schering-Plough
MGi-114 (NSC# 683863) Phase II Study
Proteasome inhibitors
Panorex (antibody 17–1A)—Phase III trials for prevention of recurrence
vinblastine and VEGF

CTP37A

ZD1839–'Iressa,' ZD6474 and ZD6126—AstraZeneca, Inc.

Corynebacterium granulosum P40—Immunotherapy—Hugo Omar De Carli, Principal Investigator, Ph: 021-84-xxxx Centro Oncologico de Excelencia Gonnet, Buenos Aires, Argentina

TAPET(R) bacterial vector—Vion Pharmaceutical's—in phase 1 trial at NCI

Rubitecan—SuperGen—Phase II Clinical Trials in: Rapidly Recurrent Advanced Colorectal Cancer in Pittsburgh

RADIATION

stereotactic radiation therapy—Radiosurgery Center at Staten Island University Hospital at 1-800-285-xxxx
other radiation approaches

Questions about Surgery and Treatment Options for Dr. Kemeny
September 24, 2000

Dear Dr. Kemeny,

As we think about the forthcoming surgery and follow-up treatment, we have a number of questions:

1) How do you evaluate the information from Dr. Heinz Lenz regarding the very high TS expression level (22.2) of the tumor and the association of high TS levels with resistance to 5-FU? Does this information suggest that the Xeloda/Celebrex combination should be discontinued? Does it mean that you and Dr. Swanson should consider Mitomycin C or Cisplatin as opposed to FUDR for the upcoming wash? If so, Dr. Swanson may need lead time to plan.

2) Given this information, should we be thinking about trying to gain access to IMC-225 or another targeting agent (e.g. Astrozeneka's ZD1839 aka Iressa) or chemo approach? If so, how do you assess the side effects and potential risks relative to possible gains? Might IMC-225 work to break down some of the

resistance to 5-FU or other chemo? (If you think C-225 is potentially the most beneficial intervention, then we will probably need sufficient lead time to gain compassionate use.) What other interventions should be considered (e.g., Rhumab-VEGF Sugen's 5416, Endostatin, Thalidomide)? What is potentially available at Sloan that should be considered?

3) We have recollection that Dr. Schwartz at MSKCC may have indicated that Joan's tumor is resistant to CPT-11. We are not sure whether his comment was based on a pathology report or simply on the fact that she had a recurrence. Do you have any path information at Sloan indicating that the tumor is resistant. If not, would it be useful to have the tumor tested for CPT-11 resistance (i.e., a Topoisomere test).

4) We spoke with Dr. Sarah Bacus at Quantitative Diagnostics Laboratories (QDL) (925 South Route 83, Elmhurst, Illinois 60126, 630-993-xxxx x 16). She suggested that we may want to consider the Topoisomere test and a VEGF test. QDL tests tumors and can get results to us within a week of receipt of the parafin-embedded tumor and a slide. They also test for P-53 and PK-21 genes. If you think it may be at all useful for you to have such knowledge, we would like to arrange to send Joan's tumor for testing. We would need a referral and also need to know what tests you think should be done. Also, Dr. Bacus mentioned that there is another company that could test a frozen section of the tumor with different chemos to measure responsiveness. Is this something that could be useful?

5) Joan has an upcoming PET scan at Sloan on Wednesday, October 4. Can we arrange a time to discuss the results with you by telephone?

You may want to know that a pre-surgical CT scan of lungs, abdomen and pelvis is scheduled for October 13. We will forward copies to you and to Dr. Fong for post-ablation evaluation. Is there any further information that would be of use to you for post-surgical treatment. Until we hear from you, Joan will continue on the Xeloda/Celebrex protocol.

Once, again, thank you for all your consideration and efforts on our behalf.

Best Wishes,

Eric & Joan Kingson

315-682-xxxx (home); 315-430-xxxx (cell phone)

fax: 315-682-xxxx; e-mail: erkingso@xxx

NEGOTIATING THE INSURANCE SYSTEM

Joan and I were fortunate to have excellent health insurance coverage. Moreover, the insurance plan was competently administered and flexible. Even so, we spent many hours negotiating medical insurance and billing issues. We also ran into a few significant problems, mostly resolved to our satisfaction. Operating on the principle that it was harder to fix than prevent potential problems, Joan and I tried, insofar as possible, to present information to our insurer in the most convincing fashion. Recognizing that her doctors were extremely busy, Joan often drafted language for them to consider in their communications with our insurance company.

The first example is a November 4, 1999, letter to Dr. Kemeny, along with suggested language that Dr. Kemeny might use in her letter requesting the highest level of reimbursement available through our insurance. Next is a letter to Joan's primary physician, Dr. Paul Kronenberg, who under our insurance plan served as the gatekeeper for referrals and reimbursement. It, too, includes suggestions for language he might use in his letter seeking authorization. Third is a draft of a letter Joan prepared for Dr. Scalzo to send to reinforce the need to reimburse for abdominal surgery. (Although originally scheduled with Dr. X, another excellent surgeon trained in this procedure, Dr. Swanson performed surgery because Dr. X was relocating his practice). Finally, Joan drafted a letter that Dr. Scalzo used to successfully request reconsideration of a claim that was denied.

Letter from Joan to Dr. Kemeny
November 4, 1999

Dear Dr. Kemeny,

As you may recall, last year you sent a letter to our insurance company stating the need for me to receive treatment here at Sloan. The insurance company approved the request through November 30, 1999, allowing us to receive the highest level of reimbursement available through our plan (Blue Cross Blue Shield of Central New York).

Once again, we need to support the need for me to receive services under your care here at Sloan. As we understand our insurance, we must make the case that this care is absolutely essential and only available at Sloan. In order to be successful in this request for level one reimbursement, we need to avoid, as was done last year, the use of the term "experimental."

We thought it might be helpful to you if we drafted part of the text of the letter. Here it is. Of course, however you write the letter will be fine with us.

Thank you, Joan Kingson

Blue Cross and Blue Shield of Central New York
Medical Services Dept.
344 South Warren Street
PO Box 4809
Syracuse, New York 13221

Re: Joan Kingson (SYU087XXXXXXX02)

Joan Kingson has been under my care during the past year for treatment of metastatic colon cancer. She has responded successfully to intervention (resection, hepatic arterial pump, and chemotherapy) for liver metastases. However, through our regular screening we have recently identified metastatic involvement in the abdomen. Based upon this early finding, I have started her immediately on what I consider to be the most efficacious chemotherapeutic treatment. This chemotherapeutic approach is not available in the Central New York region. It has much greater potential to prepare Joan for curative surgical intervention than other treatments.

Letter from Joan to Her Primary Care Physician,
Dr. Paul Kronenberg
March 24, 2000

Dear Dr. Kronenberg,

I spoke with Judy, your practice's referral specialist today about our need for authorization for 2 upcoming consultations related to resection of my abdominal metastases followed by peritoneal lavage. Dr. Kemeny, my primary medical oncologist at Sloan has recommended that we pursue this course in as timely a way as possible, given the positive response that I have had to this second chemotherapy protocol (as evidenced by the results of most recent CT and PET scans). I told Judy that we have scheduled consultations with Dr. X (March 31) and Dr. Y (April 3 or 24).

Judy is concerned about how little time there is to gain authorization. For this reason, I am drafting the following letter for you to use in any way that might be helpful. I apologize for the rush. These matters seem to have a timing of their own! I appreciate your help with this.

Sincerely,

Joan F. Kingson

Blue Cross and Blue Shield of Central New York
P.O. Box 4809
Syracuse, New York 13221

To Whomever It May Concern:

I am writing this letter on behalf of my patient, Joan King-son. For the past eighteen months, you have authorized her medical care for metastatic colon cancer by Dr. Nancy Kemeny at Memorial Sloan-Kettering Cancer Institute. Joan has responded very well to ongoing treatment for her disease, including liver resection and implantation of an hepatic pump followed by chemotherapy.

This past October, through routine CT screening, abdominal metastases were detected. At that time, you authorized continued care by Dr. Kemeny who put Joan on a promising protocol of oxaliplatin and CPT 11 with the goal of shrinking the tumor for successful resection. Joan has responded very positively to the chemotherapy (as evidenced by her most recent CT and PET scans) and it is medically necessary at this time to move toward resection of existing disease. If done in a timely manner, this intervention holds greatest potential for curative outcome.

Given the very specialized nature of this surgery, followed by peritoneal lavage, there are a very limited number of surgeons and facilities equipped to perform this intervention successfully. For this reason, it is necessary to seek care out of network. I strongly recommend that Joan consult with the two people recommended by Dr. Kemeny at this time. They are Dr. X and Dr. Y. Based upon these interviews, I recommend that she pursue surgery with the physician of her choice.

Thank you for your support and cooperation in this matter.
Sincerely,
Dr. Paul Kronenberg

Draft of Letter Prepared for Dr. Scalzo to Reinforce the Need to
Approve Reimbursement for Abdominal Surgery
May 8, 2000

Dr. Anthony Scalzo
Hematology-Oncology Associates of CNY
1000 East Genesee Street
Syracuse, New York 13210

Excellus Health Plan, Inc.
Attn: Lisa A. Antonuccio
344 South Warren Street
Syracuse, New York 13202

Dear Ms. Antonuccio:

I am writing to thank you for notification that Level One coverage has been authorized for my patient, Joan Kingson's out of area evaluation by Dr. X. As you know, I have overseen Mrs. Kingson's care for treatment of metastatic colon cancer since her diagnosis in October, 1998. Throughout this time, I have collaborated with her primary medical oncologist, Dr. Nancy Kemeny of Memorial Sloan-Kettering Cancer Center. We are very pleased with Mrs. Kingson's response to aggressive chemotherapeutic and surgical treatment.

I spoke recently with Dr. Kemeny about Mrs. Kingson's progress and planning for future treatment. At the time, she told me that she had spoken with Dr. X, subsequent to Mrs. Kingson's consultation with him. After clinical examination and review of Mrs. Kingson's reports and film, Dr. X determined her eligibility for abdominal surgery, inclusive of peritoneal lavage. He recommended that this take place in late June. Since Dr. X is in process of moving his practice, this would provide sufficient time for him to set up as well as for Mrs. Kingson to prepare for such surgery.

I strongly recommend your support of Level One coverage for this course of treatment. As I have indicated previously, this is precisely the direction Dr. Kemeny and I have been working toward since October, 1999 when disease was identified in Mrs. Kingson's abdomen. At the time, Mrs. Kingson began aggressive chemotherapy with the goal of tumor shrinkage and subsequent surgery. Based upon the results of recent scans, the tumor has responded to this chemotherapy and it is now time to move toward the treatment with greatest potential for long-term benefit.

This is a standard, yet highly specialized approach to metastatic disease in the abdomen. It is very important that Mrs. Kingson seek care from a surgeon who has successfully treated similar cases of peritoneal involvement and who is able to deliver a chemotherapeutic lavage which is compatible with her prior and ongoing adjuvant therapy. Dr. Kemeny has done considerable investigation of this approach and has located a very limited number of surgeons and sites currently equipped to deliver this service. Unfortunately there are none within this region of care. Dr. X is a highly respected and experienced professional in this area of specialization.

Once again, I thank you for taking time to consider this request. Based upon Mrs. Kingson's successful response to aggressive treatment thus far, I strongly recommend this course as the one with greatest potential for long term benefit.

Sincerely,

Dr. Anthony J. Scalzo, M.D.

Draft of an Appeal of the Insurance Company's Denial of Coverage
September 25, 2000

Excellus Health Plan, Inc.
Attn: Customer Service Department
344 South Warren Street
Syracuse, NY 13202

To Whom It May Concern:

I am writing this letter of grievance on behalf of my patient, Joan Kingson. Ms. Kingson underwent specialized abdominal surgery for colon cancer this past July. The plan granted her Level One benefits for care rendered by Dr. Richard Swanson at the University of Massachusetts Medical Center. She recovered extremely well with minimal complications.

It seems that only her initial consult of June 8, 2000 with Dr. Swanson was denied coverage at Level One. I would appreciate your reconsideration of this decision based on two points. Firstly, you granted Ms. Kingson Level One benefits for an "Out of Area Evaluation" with Dr. X in May of 2000. The consultation with Dr. Swanson was structured to evaluate my patient for precisely the same intervention considered by Dr. X. Secondly, this consult with Dr. Swanson was a requisite step toward Ms. Kingson's July surgery which you covered at Level One.

I thank you for taking time to reconsider your initial decision on this matter.

Sincerely,
Anthony J. Scalzo, MD

SEEKING ACCESS TO EXPERIMENTAL TREATMENTS

Elsewhere in this book, I mentioned that we contacted a number of researchers seeking access to experimental treatments and found, in most cases, that they were responsive and sometimes went out of their way to help. Below are several communications in which we sought to gain access to experimental treatments. First, there is an e-mail we sent to Dr. Anton Bilchik, typical of the e-mail sent to several other people who responded that Joan might be a candidate for his treatment. Next, there is a letter from Dr. Heinz Lenz who, in response to our e-mail, went out of his way to arrange for Joan's tumor to be tested at the expense of his laboratory. Third, I have included a memo I sent my friend George Igel listing all the experimental treatments I had researched and summarizing a number of telephone discussions with researchers and personnel of some pharmaceutical companies. There is a letter to Dr. Harlan Waksal, then Imclone' medical director, seeking access to C-225 (Erbitux), and finally, a letter to Dr. Scalzo thanking him for scheduling Joan's treatment with C-225.

Query about Eligibility for an Experimental Treatment

To: BilchikA@xxx
Date: Monday—July 3, 2000 2:32 P.M.
Re: Inquiry about C-Vax for my wife

Dear Dr. Bilchik,

Dr. Nancy Kemeny gave us your name and suggested we contact you about whether the C-VAX vaccine might be helpful for my wife, Joan. We can be reached at 315-430-xxxx (cell phone) or 315-682-xxxx (home); erkingson@xxx or erkingso@xxx. Dr. Kemeny's number is 212-639-xxxx in case you wish to contact her.

Joan is 48 years old and in "good health" except for the cancer. She continues to walk 2–3 miles a day and her spirits remain strong. She is scheduled to have surgery on July 17.

Joan was diagnosed with stage IV colon cancer after a hemicolectomy in Syracuse NY in October 1998. She underwent a liver resection and implantation of a HAI pump in early December 1998, followed by 6 months of chemotherapy (CPT-11 systemically and FUDR via the pump) beginning in February 1999.

She was rediagnosed with metastases in the omentum and pelvis in October, 1999. Dr. Kemeny put her on systemic oxaliplatin/cpt-11 from November to March with the goal of moving her toward a peritoneal surgery and Mitomycin C wash. Her tumors responded reasonably well and she became a candidate for surgery. Since March and until this week Joan was on Xeloda and Celebrex, which she has gone off in preparation for surgery on July 17 with Dr. Richard Swanson at University of Massachusetts Medical Center in Worcester, MA.

If you think that she may a candidate for your vaccine, please let us know whether we should make arrangements to get a tumor sample to you or whatever else we might need to do. Thank you for taking the time to review this request.

Sincerely yours,

Eric Kingson

8278 Glen Eagle Drive

Manlius, NY 13104

Response from a Cancer Researcher

From: "Lenz, Heinz"

To: erkingso@xxx

Date: Tuesday—August 22, 2000, 8:17 P.M.

Mr Kingson, thank you for your e-mail. A couple of thoughts, the test for TS gene expression makes only sense when there is reason to believe that 5-FU may still have efficacy. If there is evidence that the tumor grew under 5-FU or Xeloda, then we know that TS or related enzymes are high. If there is any doubt about this, send us a paraffin embedded tissue section (unstained) and I will ask Kathy Danenberg if she is able to run the test (the test will become available very soon as a commercial test). In addition, you should look into treatment options with cetuximab [c-225] in combination with CPT-11 which may be available at MSKCC or the PS341 trial at MSKCC.

Sincerely

Heinz-Josef Lenz

*Memo to George Igel Assessing Options for Gaining
Access to Experimental Drugs*

George,

I've done some research on drugs and on the compassionate use process. I spoke with Mike Edwards (301-496-xxxx), a pharmacist at the FDA. He will get back to me about whether there are any drugs in the FDA pipeline that might be of interest to us. He will also find out about how we might get drugs from the FDA if they have not, as yet, been approved for compassionate use. I've learned:

• The FDA keeps some drugs that are in the IND (investigational new drug) process and can make them available for compassionate use.

• If a drug is under a company initiated study and in phase III (possibly phase II) and not in the IND process, then I believe the companies are often more free to make them available than they let on. Sometimes they hold the drug back because they do not feel they have enough good results to justify release. Other times, they might not have sufficient supply.

• The FDA holds the IND for a new RAS P53 Vaccine (ADENO P53); PANOREX (ANTIBODY 17IA); ALVAC VACCINE, FOWLPOX VACCINE. For various reasons (mainly because it's too early to tell whether they will have an effect) they are not releasing these vaccines for compassionate use. However, it sounds as if it *might* be possible to get them if Dr. Kemeny felt strongly that it was worth trying them.

• The other drugs of interest are not held by the FDA and so it is possible that the companies could release them directly to Dr. Kemeny (though this might take some effort.)

My instincts are that in addition to asking her about Dr. Welt's, Dr. Schwartz's and Dr. Fong's studies, we should ask Dr. Kemeny about whether we should try to gain compassionate use of the following drugs. [To avoid repetition, I have not reproduced the entire list.]

VACCINES

CEA VAC vaccine combined with Interlekin 2—Dr. Foon (513-584-xxxx) has a trial that has begun, but is unable to add more patients because the pharmaceutical company that supplies Interleukin 2 is not providing the drug. There is a reasonable chance that Joan could be eligibile for this study after her surgery. CEA VAC (Titan Pharmaceuticals—650-244-xxxx) is going into a phase III study sponsored by the National Cancer Institute and run by the American College of Surgeons Oncology Group. However, Joan is not eligible for this. Seems like best bet is to see whether Joan could enter CEA VAC/Interlekin 2 trial. Spoke with Susan Burton again (650-244-xxxx) from Titan Pharm about the possibility of getting this through compassionate use. She said that because they do not have efficacy data, they can't to go to the FDA and make a case for opening up access for compassionate use. Also, there is no possibility of purchasing this outside the country even though it is in trial in the UK (same trial as they are opening up here). However, one route to consider is a direct plea to the CEO. Asked about whether a call from a senator might help. Got the sense that it might. It is possible to write a compassionate use protocol for one person.

CancerVax—*Dr. Anton Bilchik*—*John Wayne Medical Center*—Phase II—requires trips to California every two weeks for several months, then once a month for a year, then somewhat less frequently—Could do, but would want to know if it made sense to do Maria Gonzalez—Coordinator—310-449-xxxx (449-xxxx fax) Spoke with Ms. Gonzalez. Can only be done at John Wayne. Non-toxic. Study has been going since 1997.

Dr. Fong's study

Anti-gastrin vaccine (a.k.a. Gastrimmune)—Aphton and Aventis Pasteur collaboration Phase III neutralizes hormones (G17 & gly-extended G17)—570-839-xxxx (Aventis Pasteur) or Aphton 1-305-374-xxxx Phase III for colorectal may start in a few months. Spoke with Jeannette Whitman—305-374-xxxx (direct line) Discusssed compassionate use. Seemed interested when I asked if a request from a Senator might help. Is checking with CEO. Study suggests a significant survival advantage. Jeannette Whitman called back and said she spoke with her CEO, Mr. Phillip Gevas. Did not think it would be good to try through the FDA, but he is willing to consider making the drug available to Joan if she is able to travel to the U.K. to receive the shots. Dr. Kemeny would need to call Mr. Gevaso. She should call Jeanette Whitmore's direct line (305-374-xxxx).

Avicine Vaccine—*BIOPHARMA, INC.* (Nasdaq: AVII, AVIIW, AVIIZ), multicenter phase III trial for colorectal cancer starting in 2000 503-227-xxxx first line vaccine??? Spoke with Wendy Redhouse. David Berger, CEO—206-285-xxxx

MONOCLONAL ANTIBODIES

Dr. Welt's studies—Joan is not eligible for the one for which her tumor was tested. However, she may be eligible (if bilirubin goes down) for the other study that he mentioned (I believe this involves a chemo that tries to boost the immune system, followed by a chemo cocktail that Dr. Kemeny put together (Carmustine, 5FU, Vincristine & Streptozoci ????)

C-225—*Cetuximab*—*Imclone Dr. Harlan Waksal*—head of research 908-218-xxxx 646-638-xxxx mille van ness, clinical coordinator 908-541-xxxx, DR. XX 212-645-xxxx, Medical Director—FDA says it's an interesting drug

ANTIANGIOGENESIS

Angiostatin—Entremed, Inc.—New trial beginning. Also Endo-statin University of Wisc—Cancer Connect Line provides info on Endostatin—1-800-622-xxxx, 608-262-xxxx; also contact M.D. Anderson Info Line 1-800-392-xxxx (select option 3). Dana Farber has a company sponsored trial—617-632-xxxx (www.endostatin.dfci.harvard.edu:444/index.shtml).

SU5416—Maybe useful if we could gain compassionate use of SU5416 and combine with other chemotherapy

SU6668—Joan is on list for SU6668 phase 1 trial—However, it is only being given by itself.

IMC-1C11—Imclone has a new phase 1 colorectal cancer trial chimerized monoclonal antibody that was developed to inhibit tumor growth by preventing the development of capillaries to tumors from pre-existing blood vessels. This is accomplished by preventing a Vascular Endothelial Growth Factor (VEGF) from binding to its endothelial cell receptor (KDR). Dr. Harlan Waksal—head of research 908-218-xxxx, 646-638-xxxx mille van ness, clinical coordinator 908-541-xxxx

rhuMAb-VEGF, or anti-VEGF, in combination with chemotherapy—Genentech, Inc.—Susan D. Hellmann, M.D., M.P.H., Gen-entech's chief medical officer/ Planning phase III trial—Physicians and people with colorectal cancer inter-ested in anti-VEGF clinical trials should call 1-888-662-xxxx. Spoke with Harry Hersh (888-662-xxxx). Will have phase II trial at end of summer, but only for people who have not had chemo. Phase III may begin in December. Phase II results (104 patients)—Low dose (5 mg per kilo-gram) of Anti-Vegf—40% response rate (stable or shrink-age)/ High dose and 5fu—24%/ 5fu and leuc—17%. Does not have compassionate use program, but once phase III begins it might be possible.

RADIATION

stereotactic radiation therapy—Radiosurgery Center at Staten Island University Hospital at 1-800-285-xxxx
other radiation approaches

Letter to Imclone's Medical Director, Seeking Access to C-225 (Erbitux)
January 17, 2001

> Dr. Harlan Waksal
> Medical Director
> Imclone
> 180 Varick Street, 6th Floor
> New York, NY
> fax 212-691-xxxx

> Dear Dr. Waksal,
> I am writing to see if there is any possibility of gaining access to C-225 for my wife, Joan Kingson who tested positive for the EGFR (+2).
> You may recall that my closest friend, Dr. George Igel, spoke with you about Joan 9 or so months ago. I also believe that Mr. X may have discussed our need with you as well.
> Regardless, please allow me to tell you about our situation.
> A few personal notes first . . . We had just moved to Syracuse when Joan was diagnosed with metastatic colon cancer. Even with this illness we have a wonderful life together with our children, mainly because Joan has worked hard throughout over two years of nearly constant chemo therapies and four surgeries to maintain the spirit of our home. We have two children, Aaron (age 18) who is about to go off to college and Johanna (age 15) who is a sophomore in high school. They have been full partners in this illness and have also managed it exceptionally well. Our home remains full of warmth and humor.
> A little bragging here about our kids . . . They have made

exceptionally good adjustments to their new school and community. When Joan was diagnosed we told them that we wanted them to feel o.k. about having fun and going on with their lives as teenagers, but did not want them to feel that they "have to be having fun." They remain close to us and concerned, but have also been able to grow from and enjoy their high school years. Their friends are very present in our home and both are doing well in demanding honors courses. Aaron has focused his energies on developing a volunteer program that has involved 80 kids from his high school in regular volunteer work at an inner-city boys and girls club. A good student, he is exceptionally well-respected at his high school and is about to be awarded a county-wide award as an "unsung hero" who exemplifies the spirit of Martin Luther King at an event that will be attended by over 2000 people. He has also put considerable energy into tennis. After failing to make the varsity team as a sophomore, he worked hard and is now scheduled to play first singles at the high school. Johanna has focused her considerable energy on her studies and on athletics. She is an outstanding student who is not the least in her brother's shadow. Since coming to Syracuse she has earned varsity letters in track and soccer, and gone twice to the New York State high school championships as a member of her high school relay teams. While she watches over us very closely and gives more verbal expression to her concerns about the illness, she, too, is able to go about the business of being a teen which includes daily arguments with her brother.

About Joan (age 49)—She is an emotionally strong, physically robust and very able person. Throughout the virtually constant treatment she has continued to walk 2–3 miles nearly each day. Hence, our dog is in very good shape and I am in better shape than I would otherwise be. Joan is trained as a special education teacher and a nurse. She has many years experience working with and teaching about the needs of children and families in health care settings. Prior to our move to Syracuse, she taught child development courses for ten years at Wheelock College and coordinated a masters degree program that trained students to work in child development roles in pediatric settings. Just before we left, she completed a nursing degree at Boston College where she gradated summa cum laude.

As mentioned, we had just moved to Syracuse when Joan was diagnosed. In accepting a tenured professorship at the School of Social Work (with a secondary appointment at the Maxwell School) my largest concern was whether the transition would be smooth for Joan. This was obviously a large decision for our family and Joan was giving up a secure position at Wheelock. Little did I know what a "relatively small worry" that was. (One thing this type of illness does is put many things in perspective.)

Joan has many accomplishments, but her (and I also have to honestly assess my) greatest contribution has been living through illness and maintaining our home and watching our children grow in this period. Whatever the future brings, we are confident that they are kind people, competent and heading in the right direction and that they have the ability to handle life's ups and downs. That's about as much as we can hope for our children. And it is very much a result of Joan's working to keep us all going as we adjusted to our changed circumstances.

Well, Dr. Waskal, I am sorry to burden you with all this background but I wanted you to have a sense of who we are and why we would like to gain access to C-225, hoping it may be able to fight back this disease for awhile.

Now for the medical background . . . Joan was diagnosed with metastatic colon cancer in October 1998 after a hemi-colectomy in Syracuse, NY. We have had outstanding health care in Syracuse, New York City and Worcester Massachusetts. Her primary oncologist is Dr. Nancy Kemeny at MSKCC and her secondary oncologist is Dr. Anthony Scalzo at Hematology-Oncology in Syracuse, NY.

Joan's liver was resected at Sloan and an HAI pump implanted on 12/98. Her first chemo was systemic CPT-11 & FUDR in the pump 1/99–6/99. She was rediagnosed with peritoneal involvement in October 1998 and began systemic Oxaliplatin and CPT-11 from 11/99–3/00 in hope that it would move her toward being resectable. This was followed by Xeloda and Celebrex from mid April 2000 through early July. On July 17 her peritoneal tumors were resected/debulked in a 12 hour surgery by Dr. Richard Swanson at UMass Medical Center in Worcester, Massachusetts during which there was a heated Mitomycin C wash. Again, this was followed by Xeloda and Celebrex. In September she underwent a RFA of a liver metastasis. She was scheduled for follow-up surgery with Dr. Swanson in October 2000, but a follow-up scan showed that there was involvement in her liver and lung, rendering surgery inappropriate. In late October, Dr. Kemeny moved her to the CPT-11/5FU/Leucovoran combination (plus Celebrex). This chemo may have held the abdominal and lung involvement somewhat in check, but a recent scan indicated that there is more serious liver involvement. Hence Dr. Kemeny decided to infuse the liver directly with FUDR while continuing systemic chemotherapy. Joan is handling this chemo fairly well, but she and I have the sense that C-225 could be of greater systemic benefit, a view we believe Dr. Kemeny shares.

Well, thank you for reviewing this lengthy letter. Kindly give me a call on our cell phone (315-430-xxxx). If appropriate and convenient for you, Joan and I would also be willing to meet with you in NYC or at Imclone's New Jersey office to discuss options for gaining access to C-225.

Sincerely yours,

Eric Kingson

8278 Glen Eagle Drive

Manlius, New York 13104

Cell phone—315-430-xxxx

Thanks to Dr. Scalzo for Scheduling New Treatment

Fax To: Dr. Scalzo

From: Eric Kingson (374-xxxx—cell; 682-xxxx—home)

Date: April 4, 2001

Re: Joan

Thanks for calling us. We appreciate your taking the time to go through the options with us, especially at such a late hour. Also, thanks for moving the C-225 protocol so quickly through the IRB and for your efforts to get this drug for Joan.

I faxed a note to Dr. Kemeny. Here are some of our remaining questions.

Questions about Chemotherapy

In advance of moving on to C-225 would it be useful to use FUDR or some other drug through the pump to try to stabilize disease?

Could the pump be used with C-225? Might a low dose (or regular dose) of FUDR through the pump be advisable along with C-225 and a systemic chemo. Might C-225 potentiate the chemo through the pump? How risky would this be? Might CPT-11 through pump or some other drug be worth trying?

Should C-225 be used with CPT-11? At a regular or low dose? Is there reason to think that a lower dose of CPT-11 might be effective?

Is there any other chemo that might be useful to consider with C-225?

Other Questions

Is a second opinion regarding kidney procedure advisable? Any other tests?

At some point, might it be useful to consult with Dr. Swanson (or Dr. Fong) about surgical options to deal with symptoms and other problems related to the abdominal tumors?

Final Note of Appreciation to Readers and Acknowledgments

🎵 This is an intensely personal book. In many places emotionally wrenching to write, it must be similarly difficult for many to read—especially those facing their own or a loved one's life-challenging illness.

Some of you have similar stories and are facing parallel fears such as Joan's, of leaving what you so value, or mine, of being left. Some of you, having come uncomfortably close to finitude, may be relieved to see the promise of your or your loved one's path stretching out for many more years. Still other readers are health care professionals and students who, with your own human challenges, are also committed to helping others with theirs. You may be concerned with how to present difficult diagnoses to patients, how to engage family members, how to present hopeful treatment options, or how to say good-bye to people whose care has brought you close to their and their families' humanity. Whoever you are, I appreciate the time and emotion you gave to reading *Lessons from Joan*. Thank you. I hope your journeys lead you well.

In closing this book, I would like to share a few more thoughts and feelings. And I would like to acknowledge the assistance of many people.

I am proud to have written *Lessons from Joan*. Proud, especially, because I think I have done justice to Joan's spirit and her legacy of kindness, courage, and humor. I am a bit surprised that I finished this book. Surprised that it took form over the five summers following Joan's death, even though I was sometimes in a daze, feeling I was just writing it because I had started.

As an academic, I have authored/edited eight books, but none were so important to me as this. I was Joan's coach and advocate for three years, fully engaged in trying to protect our lives together and, with her, our children's lives. With her death, I lost Joan as well as the caregiver role that had become so central in my life. I was very sad; my kids would say very depressed.

Writing this book provided a way to continue in close relationship to Joan and reflect upon all that had happened and its meaning. It was very satisfying to complete, during the first summer, the chapter about our lives before cancer. I recall saying to myself that even if I do not finish the book, this chapter is something I wanted for Aaron and Johanna. By the second summer's end, as I completed first drafts of chapters 3, 4, and 5—the stories of diagnosis through treatment—I realized the book would probably be written.

Unlike other books I have written, I was not very concerned with its publication. I had begun writing for myself and, as I saw it, for Aaron and Johanna and other family members and friends. I certainly wanted it to be published and read by many people; only, by then, I realized the process of its writing had become more important for me than the product. The writing was providing a means of reviewing the connections between my past, present, and future and of seeking, sometimes finding and conveying, meaning from the suffering our family had experienced.

By the third summer's close, I had completed drafts of the chapters I wanted to write for myself, family, and friends; that is, everything was drafted except the appendices. These sections were finished during the fourth summer when I reorganized and revised the book, after Syracuse University Press offered to publish it.

Now in the fifth summer, as the book moves toward fall publication, there is little more to do but respond to editorial suggestions and to reflect on experiences leading to its writing. *Lessons from Joan* is far better than I thought it would be or than I could have done by myself. The ideas, suggestions, and encouragement of many make it so. Most important, it gives expression to much of what I learned from and with Joan. Coauthor of the path of our lives together since meeting in 1977, Joan is both inspiration and unseen collaborator in its writing.

I want to thank many people who helped move this book forward.

My dear friend George Igel first suggested writing about Joan and our experience of negotiating cancer and the health care system. Later, he cheered me forward. Early on when I was not sure whether I would continue with the project, I sent, at George's suggestion, beginning chapters to another grade school friend and author, John Jiler. After reviewing the manuscript, John told me he saw it as a love story waiting to be written. His comment provided motivation at that crucial time. Nick Taylor, then president of the Authors Guild and coauthor with Sidney Winawer of *Healing Lessons,* was kind enough to respond to an e-mail from me, then a total stranger. He read chapters from an early draft and provided important encouragement and advice. Three friends—health educator Helen Osborne, sociologist John Williamson, and social worker Paul Wilson—read early drafts and gave me important first feedback that helped me reflect on what I wanted to achieve in writing *Lessons from Joan.* Historian friend Andy Achenbaum read a later draft, and his enthusiasm provided momentum toward completion. The book benefited from philosopher Rick Moody's kind response to my grief when he sent selected poems of Jalal ad-Din Rumi, a thirteenth-century Sufi sage.

Family—Aaron and Johanna, Catherine Fernbach, Mary Jo Fernbach Veling, Dennis and JoEllen Fernbach, Robert and Ann Louise Fernbach, Stephen and Sophie Kingson—read portions of the manuscript, sometimes at considerable discomfort because their pain was still so present. They provided honest feedback. My kids' strong and appropriate opposition to some of what I revealed led me to make important changes. Friends—Rich Arenberg, Faith and Jonathan Ball, Howie and Madelyn Baum, Alejandro Garcia, Lou Glasse, Marcia Hartley, Gary Leavitt, Eileen Lux, Linda Butler Masters, Michele Melville, Suzanne Mendelssohn, Deborah Monahan, Gayle Mosher, Stefi Rubin, Judy Salsich, and others—worked their way through portions, sometimes painfully, and were kind to provide feedback. Dr. Nancy Kemeny and Dr. Tony Scalzo were kind enough to review the manuscript as were social workers Ann Cross and Gussie Sorensen.

Maria Brown, my graduate assistant at Syracuse University's School of Social Work, was one of the first people to read through the entire manuscript. Her corrections and other editing suggestions, conceptual and otherwise, were very helpful. Even more appreciated, her enthusiasm for the book, based in part on her experience as a breast cancer survivor, also helped move the project to completion. I would be remiss, too, if I did not acknowledge the support and generosity of the Syracuse University community, including virtually all colleagues and staff at its School of Social Work and especially Alejandro Garcia, Keith Alford, Ken Corvo, Debbie Freund, Rachael Gazdick, Rob Keefe, Bruce Lagay, Peg Miller, Deborah Monahan, Nancy Mudrick, Lisa Parker, Francis Parks, Claire Rudolph, and Carrie Smith. The assistance and thoughtful comments of Linda Thomas and Beth Sotherland, secretaries at the School of Social Work, and of Joan Bardeen, Maribeth Schoeneck, and Michael Gargan, staff for the Electronic Publishing Center, are also gratefully acknowledged.

This book is more alive and more interesting because it includes words given from the hearts of Joan, Aaron, Johanna, Catherine Fernbach, Mary Jo Fernbach, Reverend Terry Culbertson, John Jiler, Sarah Lux, and Deirdre Salsich.

I'm delighted to have Syracuse University Press publish this book. An excellent academic institution, Syracuse University's culture is supportive of employees and students. Joan and I were very grateful for the institutional and personal support of colleagues, staff, and students that facilitated our journey. Faced with the enthusiasm for the book at Syracuse University Press—especially from Mary Selden Evans, D. J. Whyte, Therese Walsh, and Peter Webber—it was immediately clear that the press would provide the right home for the book. Moreover, much of the story takes place in Syracuse, New York, and it seemed fitting that the story be published with the university's imprint. I have not been disappointed. The book has been handled with great care and professionalism. Mary Peterson Moore, manager of design and production, and her department designed a cover that wonderfully represents Joan's character. Managing editor John Fruehwirth and marketing director Theresa Litz skillfully advanced the book through the work of their departments. The copy editing of Kay Steinmetz and Ann Youmans and the proofreading of Nancy Hayes are very appreciated. And, simply put, working with Mary Selden Evans, executive editor and new friend, has been terrific.

I owe a special debt of gratitude to Carol Napoli, a nurse with deep insight and leadership experience in hospice care and grief counseling, who carefully criticized the manuscript. The final manuscript very much reflects Carol's suggestions for reorganization. Both Carol and Susan Taylor-Brown, a former Syracuse University colleague and now a professor of pediatrics at the University of Rochester Medical School, were forthright in their concerns, even where they risked opening the wounds I, and others, might prefer to avoid. I have not done all they asked, but this book is much better for their honesty and insight.

I also want to acknowledge with appreciation the generosity of Karen Davis in authoring the foreword to *Lessons from Joan*. President of the Commonwealth Fund and the first woman to head a U.S. Public Health Service agency, her many public policy, research, and scholarly contributions greatly influence the nation's health care policy discussions. For many years, I have respected her as an outstanding scholar who is deeply committed to providing access to quality health care for all Americans, especially those at greatest risk. From discussions about *Lessons from Joan*, I have learned that her intellect is fully matched by her compassion, a powerful combination.

No doubt there are some errors in this book. They are all mine. I have presented my feelings and recollections as accurately as I can. A few names have been omitted, a couple who requested anonymity and a few because I did not feel it was proper to identify them by name. Without introducing a significant change in the story, I have changed information in two places to maintain confidentiality.

There are many others—some named in the book and some not—

for whom Joan felt and I feel much gratitude for their friendship, care, and kindness. The list is long and, even at my most obsessive best, I could not provide a full accounting. Please know—whether you find your name within these pages or not—you are part of this story and appreciated.

Finally, I want to acknowledge with deepest appreciation the inspiration for this book. It comes from the kind and compassionate care Joan received. It comes from Joan's love and courage and capacity to grow, even as death approached. It comes from her determination to prepare Aaron, Johanna, and her other loves to live good, full lives. And it comes from a place beyond words, where campfires glow at water's edge.

July 16, 2005

Eric R. Kingson is professor of social work at Syracuse University's School of Social Work. He also holds a courtesy appointment as professor of public administration at the Maxwell School of Citizenship and Public Affairs. His books and other publications address political, economic, and ethical questions arising from the aging of America. A former staff adviser to two presidential commissions and a founding board member of the National Academy of Social Insurance, he is actively engaged in contemporary policy discussions about the future of Social Security and related retirement and health care policies. He and Joan were married for twenty-two years. They have two children, Aaron and Johanna.